# Adolescent Substance Abuse

## A Guide to Prevention and Treatment

## THE CHILD & YOUTH SERVICES SERIES:

EDITOR-IN-CHIEF

JEROME BEKER, *Director and Professor, Center for Youth Development and Research, University of Minnesota*

- *Institutional Abuse of Children & Youth,* edited by Ranae Hanson
- *Youth Participation & Experiential Education,* edited by Daniel Conrad and Diane Hedin
- *Legal Reforms Affecting Child & Youth Services,* edited by Gary B. Melton
- *Social Skills Training for Children and Youth,* edited by Craig W. LeCroy
- *Adolescent Substance Abuse: A Guide to Preventin and Treatment,* edited by Richard Isralowitz and Mark Singer
- *Young Girls: A Portrait of Adolescence,* by Gisela Konopka
- *Residential Group Care in Community Context—Interaction and Change: Implications of the Israeli Experience,* edited by Zvi Eisikovits and Jerome Beker

# Adolescent Substance Abuse

## A Guide to Prevention and Treatment

Richard Isralowitz and Mark Singer
Editors

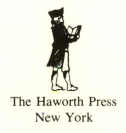

The Haworth Press
New York

*Adolescent Substance Abuse: A Guide to Prevention and Treatment* has also been published as *Child & Youth Services,* Volume 6, Numbers 1/2, Spring/Summer 1983.

The Haworth Press, Inc., 28 East 22 Street, New York, NY 10010

**Library of Congress Cataloging in Publication Data**
Main entry under title:

Adolescent substance abuse.

"Has also been published as Child & youth services, volume 6, number 1/2, spring/ summer 1983"—T.p. verso
Includes bibliographical references.
1. Youth—United States—Drug use—Prevention—Addresses, essays, lectures. 2. Youth—Drug use—Treatment—United States—Addresses, essays, lectures. 3. Substance abuse—United States—Prevention—Addresses, essays, lectures. 4. Substance abuse—Treatment—United States—Addresses, essays, lectures. I. Isralowitz, Richard. II. Singer, Mark, 1941- .
[DNLM: 1. Substance abuse—In adolescence. 2. Substance abuse—Prevention and control. Wl CH644 v.6 no.1/2 /WM 270 A2396]
HV5824.Y68A32 1983 362.2'9 83-13015
ISBN 0-86656-185-4

# Adolescent Substance Abuse: A Guide to Prevention and Treatment

Child & Youth Services
Volume 6, Numbers 1/2

## CONTENTS

# Adolescent Substance Abuse

## A Guide to Prevention and Treatment

# Introduction:
# Understanding Adolescent
# Substance Abuse

Mark Singer
Richard Isralowitz

Current studies suggest that anywhere between 20 and 40 percent of high school students use alcohol or drugs excessively (Rachal et al, 1982; Donovan and Jessor, 1978). By their senior year of high school, 90 to 95 percent of students will have experimented with some type of drug or alcohol (Braucht, 1980). Moreover, a high proportion of young people who try illicit drugs remain users (Kandel, 1982).

While the causes of adolescent substance abuse are complex and, as yet, not fully understood, its consequences are somewhat less obscure. The pervasive effects of teenage alcohol and drug abuse are not discriminatory. The psychosocial and physiological results of chemical dependency are manifest in adolescents regardless of gender, socioeconomic status, ethnicity, or area of residence. Clearly, substance abuse is one of the most serious health hazards confronting our youth.

Adolescents are at particular risk from the effects of mood altering substances. Adolescent drug/alcohol use can have more serious repercussions than adult use. The average teenager weighs less than the average adult. Since the effects of mood altering substances vary by body weight, a teenager consuming the same amount of alcohol or drugs as an adult would probably be affected to a greater extent. This is particularly problematic with respect to alcohol use because evidence suggests that youth drink less regularly than older people,

Mark Singer is affiliated with Case Western Reserve University and is in the Department of Pediatrics, Cuyahoga County Hospital, Cleveland, OH 44109. Dr. Isralowitz is in the Department of Social Work at Ben-Gurion University, Beer-Sheva, Israel. Requests for reprints should be sent to Mark Singer.

*1*

but tend to consume larger quantities per drinking occasion (Harford and Mills, 1978). Furthermore, teenagers have not yet learned to compensate for the effects of alcohol/drugs on their behaviors. This failure to compensate, combined with the many new tasks and skills learned during adolescence, makes it exceptionally difficult to behave appropriately and to perform safely while under the influence of mood altering substances.

Tragically, traffic accidents are the leading cause of death among American youth (Comptroller General of the U.S., 1979). Research has consistently demonstrated that between 45 and 60 percent of all fatal traffic accidents involving a young driver are alcohol related (U.S. Department of Health and Human Services, 1981). Finally, a developing young body is less capable of adjusting to the physical and psychological insults of alcohol/drugs than a mature body. Physical and emotional damage caused by mood altering substances are believed to occur more quickly in teenage abusers than in their adult counterparts (Finn and O'Gorman, 1981; Alibrandi, 1978).

## PURPOSE OF THE ISSUE

Due to the prevalence and effects of teenage drug and alcohol use, interest in adolescent substance abuse has increased dramatically over the past decade. As a direct consequence of this interest, services for chemically dependent youth have expanded and research in the field of adolescent substance abuse has enjoyed a revitalization. While these factors have certainly had an appreciable impact on our understanding of chemical dependency among youth, many areas of inquiry are yet to be adequately explored. It is the purpose of this issue to encourage such exploration by presenting articles which lend a new perspective to the field of adolescent substance abuse or discuss topics which have received too little attention in the literature.

## CONCEPTUAL MODELS

In all areas of human services, the manner in which we conceptualize a problem has a direct bearing upon our treatment models and therapeutic outcomes. This, of course, holds true for the field of chemical dependency. Within this field, new and competing conceptual models must emerge in order to test our present knowledge and to provide fertile ground for innovation. We have not as yet reached the point where we can be satisfied with the state of the art. Rather than reifying the current conceptual frameworks, we must constructively criticize them, and through such criticism, set the stage for the emergence of models with more explanatory power and greater treatment utility.

In the first article, Arthur Blum and Mark Singer discuss adolescent substance abuse as a manifestation of social deviance. They question whether substance abuse should be so completely partialized from other behavioral dysfunctions that theories and practices in areas such as mental health and delinquency remain largely ignored. To address this issue, the authors develop a youth assessment framework to provide a systematic means of linking a wide variety of theories to specific treatment strategies.

In his article, "Childhood: Setting the Stage for Addiction," David Sedlacek reviews the physical and psychosocial factors which predispose children to addiction. The author introduces the term "intrapsychic addiction" to describe the substrate of externally manifested addictive disorders and uses this concept as a basis for formulating an addiction model. Sedlacek argues that future research efforts must look beyond such factors as abstinence, physical improvement, or family improvement and introduce variables which are more sensitive to intrapsychic changes in the individual.

The next article, which was previously published as a part of a National Institute on Drug Abuse monograph, addresses the importance of peer-group strategies for the prevention of drug abuse. Ardyth Norem-Hebeisen and Diane P. Hedin review several key variables associated with the onset of problem behaviors and provide a conceptual rationale for the importance of peer-oriented prevention programs. The authors assert that peer influence is the dominant factor in many adolescents' entrance into drug abuse and other deviant behaviors.

## MINORITY AND DISABLED POPULATIONS

The nature and extent of adolescent substance abuse among this country's minority and disabled populations has not, as yet, been adequately documented. This may, in part, be due to the very nature of the investigatory process which tends to focus on large, accessible population groups in order to enhance generalizability or external validity. Studying harder-to-reach populations can be both time consuming and methodologically complex. In addition, these groups often do not have the sociopolitical influence to ensure their adequate share of investigatory and treatment resources. For these reasons, as well as others, only a small portion of the literature on adolescent substance abuse has focused on minority and disabled populations.

In her article on reducing drug use among Black adolescents, Laura Lee focuses on the family as an underutilized drug prevention resource. She reviews research findings related to adolescent drug use and the Black family, and calls for a unified national family policy. It is argued that such a policy would be a valuable asset in promoting primary drug prevention.

Denise Humm-Delgado and Melvin Delgado review the present state of knowledge with respect to substance abuse among Hispanic youth. They outline several factors which have inhibited a thorough analysis of Hispanic drug/alcohol abuse and identify salient issues to be addressed in the coming decade. The authors strongly suggest that attention be paid to culture-specific programs and delineate areas for future research, policy, and programming.

In the last article in this section, Ann MacEachron discusses the use of prescribed psychotropic drugs among the mentally retarded. She analyzes data on over 7,000 retarded adolescents to test empirically a proposed model of drug use. The findings suggest that interventions should not be limited to psychological and medical services, but should address needed changes in the individual's social environment as well.

## TREATMENT

The final paper in this issue addresses programming strategies for the treatment of adolescent alcohol/drug abuse. William Filstead and Carl Anderson describe a system of care and clinical issues which are central to the delivery of services to adolescents with alcohol/drug problems. The authors recognize the importance of adolescence as a developmental period and the implications this poses for treatment. Criteria are developed to distinguish the most appropriate level of care for the presenting clinical condition of the adolescent.

# REFERENCES

Alibrandi, T. *Young Alcoholics,* Minneapolis, Minn.: Comp Care Publications, 1978.

Braucht, G. N. Psychosocial research on teenage drinking. In F. Scarpitti and S. Datesman (Eds) *Drugs and the Youth Culture,* Beverly Hills, Cal.: Sage Publications, 1980. pp. 109-143.

Comptroller General of the United States, *Report to Congress on the Drinking Driver-What Can Be Done About It?,* Washington, D.C.: U.S. General Accounting Office, 1979.

Donovan, J. and Jessor, R. Adolescent problem drinking. *Journal of Studies on Alcohol,* 1978, *39,* 9, 1506-1524.

Finn, P. and O'Gorman, P. *Teaching About Alcohol,* Boston: Allyn and Bacon, 1981.

Harford, T. and Mills, G. Age-related trends in alcohol consumption. *Journal of Studies on Alcohol,* 1978, *39,* 207-211.

Kandel, D. Epidemiological and psychosocial perspectives on adolescent drug use. *Journal of the American Academy of Child Psychiatry,* 1982, *21,* 328-347.

Rachal, J. V., Guess, L., Hubbard, R., and Maisto, S. Alcohol misuse by adolescents. *Alcohol Health and Research World,* 1982, *6,* 3, 61-75.

United States Department of Health and Human Services, *Fourth Special Report to the Congress on Alcohol and Health,* Rockville, Md.: NIAAA, 1981.

# Substance Abuse and Social Deviance: A Youth Assessment Framework

Arthur Blum
Mark Singer

**ABSTRACT.** The authors discuss adolescent substance abuse as a manifestation of social deviance. Theories of adolescent deviance are reviewed in light of their contributions to understanding troubled youth. A youth assessment framework is developed to provide a systematic means of linking theories to specific treatment strategies.

The predominant approach to understanding and treating substance abuse has been to partialize it from other behavioral dysfunctions and analyze it as a unique social and individual problem. Some writers go even further and separate drug abuse and alcohol abuse as if they represent totally different problems. Programs and social policy, too, tend to reflect these separations. Thus, persons concerned with drug or alcohol abuse tend to focus their attention primarily on that body of theoretical literature, or those treatment technologies which emerge only from studies and practices specific to substance abusers. Theories and practices which have been developed in relation to other behavioral dysfunctions such as delinquency, depression, running away, etc., are largely ignored as we create separate theories, separate journals, and separate policies and programs.

## POSITION STATEMENT

The position which will be presented in this paper is that substance abuse among adolescents should be viewed as rule/norm violating behavior occurring during a developmental period in

Dr. Arthur Blum is in the School of Applied Social Sciences at Case Western Reserve University, Cleveland, OH 44106. Mark Singer is also affiliated with Case Western Reserve University and is in the Department of Pediatrics at Cleveland Metropolitan General Hospital. Requests for reprints should be addressed to Arthur Blum.

which the individual is undergoing considerable physiological and psychosocial change and stress and as part of the more general problem of social deviancy. Acceptance of this position opens the door to the utilization of a number of theories and intervention technologies which have been found useful in understanding and treating other behavior dysfunctions. It has implications, as well, for the organization and delivery of services.

Support for our position can be found in the reality that very few adolescent substance abusers have substance abuse as their only problem. More likely, substance abusers are also involved in other delinquent acts, or have run away, or have school problems, or are involved in a family conflict situation which has included violence or incest and on, and on. Investigators and practitioners who specialize in other areas of social deviance have, likewise, found that individuals most often reflect a multitude of rule/norm violating behavior, especially if any of the problems have gone untreated for a length of time. Unfortunately, the choice of which "specialist" will dictate the course of treatment is most often dependent on chance or who recognizes and becomes concerned about some aspect of the behaviors, not on the basis of theoretical insights or assessments. Adolescents who are in trouble may be more subject to chance events in relation to help than are the gamblers at the crap tables of Las Vegas.

Having now stated our general position, we would like to examine it more closely, with some modifications, in relation to various phases of *dealing* with the problem of social deviance in adolescence. Our focus is on the applications and, thus, throughout this paper, we will attempt to organize our discussion of theories and approaches to social deviance from the perspective of the practitioner or program planner who is responsible for "doing" something about it—who must apply knowledge—rather than from the perspective of creators of new knowledge or theory. This perspective will affect the way we have chosen to identify what knowledge is important, and for what aspects of program, to provide a framework for categorizing and screening theories which we think can be useful to the practitioner.

Programs designed to deal with deviance fall into three categories based on their desired outcomes. (A single, comprehensive program may include all three outcomes, but the approaches within the program, or parts of the program, can be subdivided.) First, there are programs whose major goals are *prevention and/or early identification* of adolescents who are at risk or are showing initial signs of behavioral problems. This program focus should not be limited in either its underlying theories or in the program design to substance abuse. Rather, they should reflect an understanding and approach to the range of rule/norm violating behavior in adolescence since there is such great overlap among behaviors.

Second, there are those programs and interventions which are aimed at stopping the problematic behaviors which we will call *acute treatment* programs. Although there seems to be some agreement in the field that the first step in the treatment of any deviant behavior is to stop the behavior, the appropriate technologies for doing this are problem specific. The design of programs for the acute treatment of drug abuse, alcoholism, stealing, running away etc., are different and must be based on knowledge which is highly specific to the particular behavior. It is in relation to acute treatment programs that we must modify our position that substance abuse should be viewed as one aspect of the general problem of social deviance in adolescence. Specialized knowledge about the particular behavior must be utilized to design acute treatment programs.

Third, once the behavior is stopped, programs and interventions must focus on *supporting and maintaining* the individual as he or she readjusts to a lifestyle free of the deviant behavior. Again, our position is that there are common factors and theoretical understandings which should dictate the design of such programs within the broader category of social deviance. Support and maintenance programs addressing the range of adolescent behavior problems should have greater similarity than difference.

Thus, the remainder of this paper will focus on the knowledge base from which practitioners should draw in developing programs whose aims are the prevention and/or early identification of social deviance or the support and maintenance of individuals who have displayed deviant behavior, including substance abuse. This approach follows the lead of Jesser et al. (1968), who propose that understanding substance abuse requires a multi-variable approach and the utilization of a wide range of knowledge about adolescent development and dysfunctional behaviors.

## ADOLESCENCE AND DEVELOPMENT TASKS

Underlying any program dealing with social deviance must be a firm knowledge of the "normal" developmental tasks of adolescents. A major question in assessment is "from what are adolescents deviating?'' Adolescence is a period of change, transition, and upheaval on the part of adolescents themselves, and it is shared by or inflicted upon the significant others around them. The turmoil is related to the crucial nature of the developmental life tasks and circumstances that face youth during this period of their lives. Focusing on the tasks, rather than the dynamics of adolescent development, has the advantage of providing for the practitioner specificity in relation to the need, the intervention, and the desired outcome.

Some of the more salient tasks include: 1) development of a system of values, beliefs and goals which will serve to guide behavior; 2) establishment of personal identity and self-image as it relates to changes in body size and shape, physical coordination, and personal perception of one's own competence and mastery in social, physical, and cognitive areas; 3) development of interpersonal skills and relationships in relation to peers of the same and opposite sex, dealing with separation from family dependency and establishing a more independent role, and dealing with non-parent adults in such realms as school, employment, leisure activities, etc.; and 4) establishing and clarifying one's goals and roles as related to occupation, sex, marriage and family, and future lifestyle. These are, indeed, formidable tasks and their pursuit, under the best of conditions, is stressful. In prevention programs, recognition of these stresses is critical and, in support and maintenance programs, we must remember that even after the dysfunctional behavior subsides, the adolescent must be helped to accomplish successfully these common growth tasks if s/he is to function appropriately.

## THEORIES OF DEVIANCE

A number of theories have been proposed for explaining adolescent deviance. Although each of them adds to our understanding, none provides a definitive explanation or usable single ''grand'' theory. Each of the theories adds some insights about a particular type or cause of deviance, but few address the issue of multiple causation and multiple types of deviance. Given that each of the theories explains some aspect of deviant behavior, a practitioner, to make good use of the available theories, must undertake an assessment process which allows him to place the individual client within the appropriate theoretical framework. Once this assessment is made, the practitioner can then utilize the different practice insights and techniques which are linked to the various theories and develop differential approaches for particular clients or client groups. Too often, the choice of intervention is made before there is an adequate assessment. We thus tend to pick a single approach with which we are familiar and comfortable without considering the range of explanations which dictate differential approaches for particular clients. It is critical that we develop a better process for systematically reviewing the many theories and factors which should be taken into consideration in designing a program or developing a plan to serve individual youth.

We have attempted to develop a typology of deviance theories based on a wide range of existing theories which we think have implications for program design and treatment. Rather than utilizing the existing groupings based on social science disciplines, we have tried to group the theories for use by practitioners. The choice of categories is based on the implications for the focal point of the intervention, i.e., institutions, peer group, family, individual, etc., the goal of the intervention and the implied technology. The typology will, hopefully, be of use for assessing both program direction and the needs of individual youth. We have not attempted an exhaustive review of all deviance theories, nor have we specified all of their treatment implications. Rather, we have tried to present a usable framework for assessment and to illustrate how it could be used for planning differential programs and interventions which meet the variety of needs of troubled youth.

We believe that, for the purposes of practice, deviance theories can be grouped into the following six categories: 1) Socialization or Value Development Theories; 2) Institutional Provision and Opportunity Theories; 3) Peer Group Theories; 4) Family Theories; 5) Personality and Self-Image Theories; and 6) Biogenic Theories.

## *1. Socialization or Value Development Theories*

Explanations of the relationship between value development and deviant behavior have been offered from a variety of perspectives, including the differences in value orientation in delinquency areas (Kobrin, 1941), the importance of differential associations (Sutherland, 1947), the effects of lower class culture (Kvaraceus and Miller, 1959) and neighborhood values (Shaw and McKay, 1942), the importance of the concept of anomie (Merton, 1949), and the theory of neutralization (Sykes and Matzo, 1957).

Emerging from this range of theoretical approaches there are three subgroups of troubled youth: 1) socialized youth whose deviant behavior must be explained by other theories; 2) unsocialized youth whose behavior is the result of the lack of internalization of values and who therefore are susceptible to situational stimuli and stress; and 3) negatively socialized youth who have a clear set of values but whose values are in conflict with those of the larger society. These sub-groups are indeed different and any program approach must be adapted to these differences.

Value development is seldom addressed directly as the focus for treatment; instead, it is usually incorporated into such concepts as self-image. The critical point in the theoretical approaches cited above is that one's social environment is the source of one's value orientation; consequently, efforts to affect a youth's values or socialization process must be directed at the environmental source as well as to the individual. Each of the theories identifies a different environmental source, thus interventions should relate to the particular environmental source which is influencing the value formation of the specified sub-group of troubled youth.

## 2. Institutional Provision and Opportunity Theory

A second group of theories explains deviance on the basis of the blockage of legitimate opportunities for success and the resulting use of illegitimate means for achieving legitimate ends (Cloward and Ohlin, 1961; Cressey, 1970), the failure of schools to provide adequate education (Polk and Schafer, 1972; GAO, 1976), the negative effects of labeling by institutions (Becker, 1963; Thorsell and Klemke, 1972), and the consistently high unemployment rates of youth. Although these theories can be grouped for classification purposes, each implies a specific but different target for intervention.

These theories call attention to the importance of institutional arrangements in the society which can make it nearly impossible for some youth to either acquire needed skills or to have effective access to employment opportunities. Existing drop-out rates in the schools, the failure of school systems to provide basic educational preparation, the failure of school systems to provide adequate vocational programs, and the persistent inability of the economic system to absorb youth into the labor market are frequently subjects of newspaper articles. More recently, they have become the basis of law suits. We must engage in efforts to bring about institutional changes that will result in more adequate educational preparation for youth, and an expansion of employment opportunities for them to prevent deviant behaviors.

However, we cannot wait for these basic institutional changes to occur in planning treatment programs for today's troubled youth. Counselors must find ways to make optimal use of available opportunities, and act as advocates for their clients with existing institutions. Effective support and maintenance programming requires that major attention be given to these obstacles to opportunity for youth, and that counselors have knowledge about and access to such existing resources as special education and job training programs. They must assume an advocacy posture in attempting to get school systems to develop needed educational programs that meet the specific needs of their clients. The theories in this grouping emphasize the need for programs to relate specifically to the educational and employment needs of youth.

## 3. Peer Group Theories

A number of theories have been based upon the observation that a significant amount of deviant behavior in our society takes place in the context of peer groups. Beginning with the classic studies of Thrasher (1936) and Whyte (1934), there has been elaboration of this school of thought with such concepts as peer subculture (Cohen, 1955; Miller, 1958; Scott and Vaz, 1963; Block and Neiderhoffer, 1958), counter-culture (Yinger, 1960), and with some indepth studies of particular types of groups (Yablonsky, 1963; Short and Strodtbeck, 1965).

The writings indicate that peer groups exert two types of influences that result in deviant behavior. First, peer groups can effectively set normative standards for the behavior of their members—they may demand conformity with group norms of deviant behavior. Second, groups can create the stimulus, contagion, and support for occasional deviant behaviors which are neither consistent with the values of individual members of the group nor represent ongoing group norms.

The importance of peer groups as a contributing factor to deviance has led to the development of approaches which utilize the peer group in prevention and treatment. It is important, however, to recognize that, as each theory specifies the particular type of influence the group exerts, the assessment must identify, and group interventions relate to different types of group influence. As indicated earlier, for one group member the group may provide a normative influence, while for another, the same group may provide contagion. An intervention must be analyzed and planned both in relation to the group and to the individual member involved. These matters must be taken into consideration when forming therapy groups where one must be clear as to the goal of the group, the appropriate intervention to achieve the goal, and the differential selection of members in light of the group goal.

## 4. Family Theories

A number of theories have been proposed which associate family variables with deviant behavior. Gleuck and Gleuck (1962) and Nye (1958) have each reviewed the most relevant of these theories. The variables which have been studied from a number of different perspectives include broken homes, single parent families, deviant behaviors of the parents, role confusion in the family, family inconsistencies in discipline and limit setting, family violence and incest, the lack of parental affection and provision, and deficient communication (for theories specific to substance abuse, see Maddox and McCall, 1964; and Zucker, 1976). While each of these variables has been found to be associated with some deviant behavior in particular studies, they apply to only a small percentage of deviant population; they offer no explanation for the large number of youth who experience similar family situations but do not become involved in deviant acts. Perhaps it is because of the established importance of the family in child development and the accessibility of some families to treatment that counselors have tended to attribute greater importance to the explanatory value of family theories than is warranted by existing evidence.

Again, interventions must be designed that rectify or compensate for the specific deficiency involved. In addition to individual and family counseling approaches, consideration must be given to the use of homemakers, Big Brothers and Big Sisters, jobs for youth, and income provision programs for independent living arrangements. Removal from the family may be indicated in the most extreme cases. Older youth often cannot wait until their family is rehabilitated. The family pattern may be so fixed or may contribute so greatly to their needs to rebel that other alternatives must be sought.

In all cases, an assessment should be made as to how well the family provides for the needs of the youth and any interventions in a youth's family life should be made on the basis of very specific treatment goals.

## 5. Personality and Self-Image Theories

Since counselors most often interact with individual youth, it is understandable that a great deal of emphasis has been placed on individually-oriented personality and self-image theories to explain deviant behavior. Psychoanalytic theory (Aichorn, 1936; Friedlander, 1947; Redl and Wineman, 1956), identity development (Erikson, 1950), learning theory (Ullman and Krasner, 1969), labeling theory (Lemert, 1967), and self-image concepts (Reckless, Dinitz and Murray, 1956; Reiss, 1951) represent only a small sample of the deviance theories based on personal psychology.

Still, we have not answered the basic question: To what extent is deviant behavior the result of internalized, self-perpetuating dynamics, as compared with external factors? Given that a youth may be responding to environmental influences, at what point do these influences, and the gratifications he receives from his behavior, affect his personality development to the point where the initial stimulus is no longer needed and the behavior itself is self-regenerating or addictive? At the same time, we must ask whether therapy can be effective if the self-regenerating aspects of the behavior are neutralized, but the initial environmental stimuli remain unchanged. We often expect that changes in an individual will prove powerful enough to equip him to withstand the pressure of the environmental forces with which he must contend. For many troubled youth, however, staying "straight," in view of the daily situational stresses they face, requires that they have individual strengths beyond those of the average person. Support and maintenance programs must keep this in mind.

Individual counselling approaches vary greatly depending upon the theories of behavior from which they are derived. These variations may be less critical than the question of whether the other variables involved in the case—values, institutions, peer groups, etc.— contribute significantly to the deviant behavior. It has been our experience that much of the failure in treating troubled youth is due to limiting interventions only to individual counselling. Counselling can be very helpful, but in many cases it must be combined with work directed toward other contributing factors.

## 6. Biogenic Factors

The debate as to the differential effects of heredity and environment rages on and, although not resolved, cannot be ignored. Studies have indicated a possible relationship between dysfunctional behavior and minimal brain dysfunction (Woods, 1961; Assael, Kohen-Ray, and Alpern, 1967), chromasomal anomaly (Court-Brown, Price, and Jacobs, 1968; Marinelli, Berkson, Edwards and Bannerman, 1969) and physical characteristics (see Rees, 1973 for review). Most recently, evidence has emerged that suggests genetic factors may have an important influence on susceptibility to alcoholism (Saunders, 1982; Bohman, 1978). Consideration must be given to special approaches to those cases which show evidence of physiological and biological genesis, as well as for cases more amenable to environmental and psychodynamic explanation.

The theories cited above are representative of the range of theories developed to explain the phenomenon (or more correctly, phenomena) of deviance. For the most part, the study samples from which these theories are drawn include males only—little attention has been paid to the degree to which they are applicable to females.

In order to be helpful to the practitioner, our categorization of the theories is based partly on specific linkages to differing focuses of treatment and to choices among the range of interventions available. The theoretical groupings tend to cut across traditional academic disciplines. The practitioner, thus, must be prepared to select the appropriate knowledge from more than one discipline to help him understand the acts of the particular individual with whom he must deal. Let us now proceed to see how this categorization of existing theories can be put to practical use in the assessment and treatment of youth.

## YOUTH ASSESSMENT FRAMEWORK

The six categories of theories indicated above can be translated into six focal points for treatment. For some youth, the treatment plan must address value development or change in values. For others, affecting societal institutions and lack of opportunities becomes crucial. And, in still other cases, peer groups, family influences, or intrapsychic conflicts should be the main concern. In cases in which there are biogenic factors at play, special programs and approaches must be developed that will at least neutralize their negative effects.

It is our contention that one reason for the relatively poor success of substance abuse programs has been a tendency to try to force all clients into a single conceptual category and to utilize a single explanation of their behavior (and a single treatment approach). Even in instances in which the investigation and diagnostic statement include a range of contributory variables, the program frequently reflects a single focus or, at best, a limited range of interventions. We tend too often to do what we know how to do—individual counseling, group counseling, etc.—even if it is not the most appropriate treatment approach for the particular case or client group.

In order to avoid reductionism, the assessment process must provide a systematic means of insuring that consideration is given to a wide range of alternative explanations. The diagnostic statement should fully reflect each individual's situation. In cases in which there are multiple causative factors at work, the treatment plan should explicitly indicate the specific approaches which will be used to modify or compensate for each of the relevant factors. Only then will we have truly adapted our treatment to the needs of youth. And, we will be in a better position to assess whether what we can offer is powerful enough to offset the pressures toward deviancy. We might also, then, be able to evaluate the reasons for our successes and failures.

We are proposing an assessment framework based on the six categories of theory. Figure I presents a matrix which can be used to assess individuals or sub-groups and to plan specific intervention. During the study process, the client or client group should be assessed in each of the six categories on the basis of the various theories within each category, to determine whether and in what ways factors related to each of the categories contribute to the problematic behavior. The assessment would provide a "problem profile" for each client or client group. These profiles could, and in our experience will, differ greatly among the client populations. For some youth, family or self-image factors may be the most critical contributing factors, while for others, peer group, value development, and institutional provision factors may be more important.

In each instance where it is determined that there is a factor within

FIGURE 1

Youth Assessment Framework

| Theories | Assessment | Treatment Plan (Specific intervention) |
|---|---|---|
| | Problem   No Problem | |

I. Value Development

II. Institutional Provision and Opportunity

III. Peer Group

IV. Family

V. Personality and Self-image

VI. Biogenic Factors

the category which is contributing to the problematic behavior, there should be a specific intervention in the treatment plan aimed at relieving, changing, or compensating for its influence. For example, negative family interactions in a particular case may be highly influential in stimulating the deviant behavior. The treatment plan should specify whether the goal is to try to change the interaction through family counseling, try to compensate for lack of family support by placing the youth in a peer support group, or try to relieve the stress by developing an alternative living situation if the family situation cannot be affected. If this same youth is also having a school problem (i.e., learning problem, truancy, etc.), the plan should also indicate the particular intervention aimed at the specific school problem and whether the goal is changing the school situation, such as transferring from an academic to a vocational program, compensating for it by tutoring, etc., or relieving the situation by finding an alternative special education or work training program. Whatever the contributing factors, the plan for the youth should specifically address it.

It is likely that in cases in which there are multiple factors, they cannot all be addressed at the same time. In these instances, the plan should outline a progression of steps and a projected time sequence that may require that we first find an alternative living arrangement, then involve the youth in a peer support group and, as he is able to utilize the peer support, design a tutoring program. The assessment framework should provide a type of checklist which both identifies the contributing factors and indicates how the treatment plan and procedures address each of them. This multiple factor approach recognizes the interrelatedness of deviant behaviors, the complexity of multifactor assessment, and the requirement for differential program and individual approaches. Programs aimed at prevention and early identification, and support and maintenance of troubled youth must encompass this range of assessment and intervention alternatives.

## A CAVEAT

It is obvious that the Youth Assessment Framework reflects a classification scheme that is neither conceptually nor theoretically elegant. The scheme is not unidimensional—it mixes the conceptual equivalents of apples, oranges, and pears. The state of present knowledge, however, does not allow a more sophisticated rendering at this time. Thus, the practitioner is faced with utilizing knowledge across various social science disciplines and organizing it for use in program design and treatment.

This framework represents a beginning attempt to try to systematize current thinking and to make linkages between theories and specific treatments. Much work remains. In particular, we must determine more clearly what the differential effects are when given treatments, e.g., individual counseling, peer group counseling, are applied to different types of cases, e.g., negative value structure, lack of opportunity, poor self-image. The road toward developing more effective treatment for troubled youth or, indeed, for any kind of specialized clientele, is formidable. It does not seem likely that we shall ever reach our humanistic and professional objectives until we more systematically engage that long and arduous journey.

## REFERENCES

Adams, J. *Understanding adolescence.* Boston: Allyn and Bacon, 1973.

Aichorn, A. *Wayward youth.* London: Putnam, 1936.

Assael, M., Kohen-Ray, R., and Alpern, S. Developmental analysis of EEG abnormalities in juvenile delinquents. *Diseases of the Nervous System,* 1967, *28,* 49-54.

Becker, H. S. *Outsiders: Studies in the sociology of deviance.* London: Free Press, 1963.

Bloch, H. W., and Niederhoffer, A. *The gang: A study of adolescent behavior.* New York: Philosophical Library, 1958.

Bohman, M. Some genetic aspects of alcoholism and criminality. *Archives of General Psychiatry,* 1978, *35,* 269-276.

Clark, J. P., and Wenninger, E. P. Social class and delinquency. *American Sociological Review,* 1962, *27,* 826-834.

Cloward, R. A., and Ohlin, L. E. *Delinquency and opportunity.* Glencoe: Free Press, 1961.

Cohen, A. K. *Delinquent boys: The culture of the gang.* Glencoe: Free Press, 1955.

Court-Brown, W., Price, W., and Jacobs, P. Further information on the identity of 47, XYY males. *British Medical Journal,* 1968, *2,* 325-328.

Craft, M., Stephenson, G., and Granger, C. A controlled trial of authoritarian and self-governing regimes with adolescent psychopaths. *American Journal of Orthopsychiatry,* 1964, *34,* 543-554.

Cressey, D. R. Organized crime and inner-city youth. *Crime and Delinquency,* 1970, *16,* 132-135.

Donovan, J., and Jessor, R. Adolescent problem drinking: Psychosocial correlates in a national sample study. *Journal of Studies on Alcoholism,* 1978, *39,* 1506-1523.

Elder, G. *Adolescent socialization and personality development.* Chicago: Rand McNally, 1968.

Erikson, E. H. *Childhood and society.* New York: W.W. Norton, 1950.

Friedlander, K. *The psychoanalytic approach to delinquency.* New York: International Universities Press, 1947.

Gallatin, J. *Adolescence and identity.* New York: Harper and Row, 1975.

Glueck, S., and Glueck, E. *Family environment and delinquency.* Boston: Houghton-Mifflin, 1962.

Glueck, S., and Glueck, E. *Of delinquency and crime: A panorama of years of search and research.* Springfield, Ill.: Charles C. Thomas, 1974.

General Accounting Office, Comptroller General of the United States. *Learning disabilities: The link to delinquency should be determined, but schools should do more now.* Washington, D.C.: U.S. Government Printing Office, 1976.

Jessor, R., Graves, T., Hanson, R., and Jessor, S. *Deviant behavior: A study of a tri-ethnic community.* New York: Holt, Rinehart and Winston, 1968.

Kandel, D. Epidemiological and psychosocial perspectives on adolescent drug use. *Journal of the American Academy of Child Psychiatry,* 1982, 21, *4,* 328-347.

Kobrin, S. The conflict of values in delinquency areas. *American Sociological Review,* 1951, *16,* 653-666.

Kvaraceus, W. C., and Miller, W. B. *Delinquent culture: Culture and the individual.* New York: National Education Association, 1959.

Lambo, T. A. Aggressiveness in the human life cycle within different sociocultural settings. *International Social Science Journal,* 1971, *23,* 79-88.

Lemert, E. *Human deviance, social problems and social control.* Englewood Cliffs, N.J.: Prentice-Hall, 1967.

Marinelli, M., Berkson, R., Edwards, J., and Bannerman, R. A study of the XYY syndrome in tall men and juvenile delinquents. *Journal of the American Medical Association,* 1969, *208,* 321-325.

Maddox, G., and McCall, B. *Drinking among teenagers.* New Brunswick, N.J.: Rutgers Center of Alcohol Studies, 1964.

Merton, R. K. Social structure and anomie. In R.K. Merton (Ed.), *Social theory and social structure.* Glencoe, Ill.: Free Press, 1949.

Miller, W. B. Lower class culture as a generating milieu of gang delinquency. *Journal of Social Issues,* 1958, *14,* 5-19.

Nye, F. I. *Family relationships and delinquent behavior.* New York: Wiley, 1958.

Polk, D., and Schafer, W. E. *Schools and delinquency.* Englewood Cliffs, N.J.: Prentice-Hall, 1972.

Reckless, W. C., Dinitz, S., and Murray, E. Self-concept as an insulator against delinquency. *American Sociological Review,* 1956, *21,* 744-746.

Redl, F., and Wineman, D. *Children who hate.* Glencoe, Ill.: Free Press, 1956.

Rees, L. Constitutional factors and abnormal behavioi. In H. Eysenk (Ed.), *Handbook of Abnormal Psychology.* London: Pittman Medical, 1973.

Reiss, A. J. Delinquency as the failure of personal and social controls. *American Sociological Review,* 1951, *16,* 196-206.

Saunders, J. Alcoholism: New evidence for a genetic contribution. *British Medical Journal,* 1982, *284,* 1137-1138.

Schoenfield, C. G. A psychoanalytic theory of juvenile delinquency. *Crime and Delinquency,* 1971, *17,* 469-481.

Scott, J. W., and Vaz, E. W. A perspective on middle-class delinquency. *Canadian Journal of Economic and Political Science,* 1963, *29,* 324-335.

Shaw, C. R., and McKay, H. D. *Juvenile delinquency in urban areas.* Chicago: University of Chicago Press, 1942.

Short, J., Jr., and Stodtbeck, F. O. *Group process and gang delinquency.* Chicago: University of Chicago Press, 1965.

Sutherland, E. H. *Principles of criminology.* New York: Lippincott, 1947.

Sykes, G. M., and Matza, D. Techniques in neutralization: A theory of delinquency. *American Sociological Review,* 1957, *22,* 664-670.

Teeters, N. K., and Reinman, J. O. *The challenge of delinquency.* New York: Prentice-Hall, 1950.

Thorsell, B. A., and Klemke, L. W. The labeling process: Reinforcement and deterrent? *Law and Society Review,* 1972, *6,* 393-403.

Thrasher, F. M. *The gang.* Chicago: University of Chicago Press, 1936.

Ullman, L. P. and Kramer, L. *A psychological approach to abnormal behavior.* Englewood Cliffs, N.J.: Prentice-Hall, 1969.

Vorrath, H. H., and Brendtro, L. K. *Positive peer culture.* Chicago: Aldine, 1974.

Wechsler, H., and Thum, D. Teenage drinking, drug use and social correlates. *Quarterly Journal of Studies on Alcohol,* 1973, *34,* 1220-1227.

Weeks, H. A. *Youthful offenders at Highfields.* Ann Arbor: University of Michigan Press, 1963.

Whyte, W. F. *Street corner society.* Chicago: University of Chicago Press, 1943.

Woods, S. Adolescent violence and homocide: Ego disruption and the 6 and 14 dysrhythmia. *Archives of General Psychiatry,* 1961, *5,* 528-534.

Yablonsky, L. *The violent gang.* New York: Macmillan, 1963.

Yinger, M. J. Contraculture and subculture. *American Sociological Review.* 1960, *25,* 625-635.

Zucker, R. Parental influence on the drinking patterns of their children. In M. Greenblatt and M. Schuckit (Eds.), *Alcoholism problems in women and children.* New York: Grune and Stratton, 1976.

# Childhood:
# Setting the Stage for Addiction

## David A. Sedlacek

**ABSTRACT.** The author begins by describing various terms that are used in discussion of addictive disorders and how they relate to one another. The term "intrapsychic addiction" is proposed as describing the substrate of the externally manifested addictions (chemical dependency, compulsive gambling, eating, overwork, etc.). The author then reviews the physical, psychological and social factors which predispose children to addiction. A model relating these various factors to one another is presented.

Many and varied terms are used in discussing problems associated with the use of alcohol, mood altering drugs and other addictive disorders. A lack of precision in both the definition and use of terms creates conceptual difficulties which impair not only our thinking about this problem but also our approach to its treatment. Problems surrounding the definition and use of terms relating to the addictive disorders are more critical in children and adolescents than in adults. Appropriate diagnosis and subsequent treatment depends upon the accurate conceptualization of a problem. While misdiagnosis is potentially harmful to an adult, the inappropriate over- or under-diagnosis of an addictive disorder in a youth can have lifelong negative implications. With the above in mind, this article will begin with a discussion of a hierarchical model of addictive disorders as they relate to alcohol and drugs in order to put frequently used terms into perspective. Various childhood factors which predispose a person to addiction will then be explored.

David A. Sedlacek is in Family Medicine at Case Western Reserve University, Cleveland, OH 44106. Requests for reprints should be addressed to the author.

## INTRAPSYCHIC ADDICTION

First of all, don't be put off by the word "intrapsychic." Here it signifies within the psyche or self. Intrapsychic addiction, then, refers simply to addiction rooted within oneself as opposed to outside of oneself. Intrapsychic addiction can be defined as the compulsive, chronic use of a self defeating pattern of thinking and behaving (including the use of mood altering chemicals) secondary to the inability of the person to make consistently healthy decisions on his or her own behalf. A relatively large segment of our population has intrapsychic addiction which has also been called a disability of the will (Culver and Gert, 1981, pp. 188-201) or a volitional disorder (Mule', 1981). A volitional disorder implies that a person is unable to reason or make use of the will to arrive at healthy personal decisions at any given moment. This concept must be clearly distinquished from the moralistic view of addiction which states, for example, in relation to alcoholism that if only the person wanted to stop drinking he would. What is being stated here is the antithesis of the moralistic approach. The concept of intrapsychic addiction implies that there is a malfunctioning of the will making it impossible for the person to make healthy choices about what is best for him or her at any given moment.

There are numerous manifestations of intrapsychic addiction. Alcohol and drug addiction are frequently mentioned, but also included in this category are compulsive eating, gambling, smoking, working, sexual activity, and a variety of other socially acceptable and unacceptable behaviors. Some authors (Love, 1978; Mule', 1981) consider these behaviors symptoms of the underlying intrapsychic addiction or volitional disorder which is in accord with this author's point of view. However, there is an inherent danger in this viewpoint making the mistake that has been made by psychiatry in its futile attempt to treat alcohol and drug addiction. The logic goes like this: If you treat the underlying symptoms (unresolved feelings about the past, depression, etc.) the alcohol or drug problem will disappear. The fallacy of this logic becomes clear when several additional factors are considered. First, there is the physical addiction which necessitates that the addicted person first stop taking the chemical. Second, the preoccupation with the addictive behavior becomes so strong that in spite of all the personal pain it causes, it will continue unless directly addressed. Third, minimization and denial of the addictive behavior makes it unlikely that it can be treated by indirect means in its initial stages.

In spite of the fact that the alcohol or drug addiction becomes the predominant or principle problem, however, it is this author's view that the alcohol or drug addiction is not the essence of the person's addiction. Even Alcoholics Anonymous describes alcoholism as a symptom of a spiritual disease (Alcoholics Anonymous, 1976, p. 64). Take a look at the very successful approach which has been developed for the treatment of chemical dependency. Very little time is spent on the physical addiction. Withdrawal symptoms are generally easily managed in two to three days. Next, the person must come to admit and then accept that a chemical dependency problem exists. This is accomplished by confrontation, personal sharing, and formal education about chemical dependency. Many programs, especially some adult programs, emphasize this educational approach and then expose their patients to the first few steps of Alcoholics Anonymous.

In addition to the philosophical problem of having professionals get paid for doing the voluntary work of A. A., there are serious therapeutic shortcomings to a predominantly educational/A. A. approach to treatment. First, not all patients are ready to meet the program's timetable for getting well (e.g., complete A.A.'s fifth step in the first 30 days). Second, even Alcoholics Anonymous tells us that its program is for those who are able to want it. *"If* you have *decided you want* what we have and are *willing* to go to any length to get it—*then* you are ready to take certain steps" (ibid, p. 58-emphasis added.). Most addicts enter treatment unwillingly. They agree to treatment because they don't want to be sick, get kicked out of school, or be forced to leave home. Few, if any, enter treatment with a positive "want to," i.e., wanting to grow as a person because they see themselves as intrinsically worth the effort. If they had possessed a healthy view of themselves and had known how to live, they probably would not have become chemically dependent. The better treatment programs recognize that helping the addict to *want to be well* is the primary task of treatment.

Once this has been accomplished, then Alcoholics Anonymous or other similar growth producing therapies can take over. Getting an addict to want to be well and giving him or her the ability to reason is not an easy task in a person who is devoid of self-love. Reactions, old thinking patterns, and an inability to deal honestly with personal feelings all stand in the way of learning how to make healthy personal decisions. The better programs recognize that learning to live, at best, only begins during the initial treatment period. Strong aftercare coupled with self-help support groups are vital to the maintenance of a chemically free and personally growthful lifestyle.

Why has so much time been taken up describing intrapsychic addiction? If we are to describe the childhood factors leading to addiction, then we must clearly know the essence of addiction. Hopefully, by doing so, we can help some young people avoid the tragedy that is seen in Alcoholics Anonymous every day—members who are not able to utilize fully the richness of the program because they don't know how very special they are as human beings.

## CHEMICAL DEPENDENCY

Another term which is used frequently is chemical dependency. This term recognizes that alcohol and other types of mood-altering drugs are all used in a dependency relationship in order to help the individual repeatedly avoid some type of intrapsychic pain. However, the field is doing itself a disservice by failing to distinguish the predominant physical and/or psychological addiction to the chemical from the intrapsychic addiction as has been described above. While it is true that the field of chemical dependency treatment has developed the prototype for dealing with both aspects of addiction, the basic principles of recovery have been successfully applied to several other psychobehavioral disorders as well (Mule', 1981). The danger is that the field of chemical dependency treatment may become too myopic in its approach. Many individuals admitted to chemical dependency treatment programs are also overweight or compulsive gamblers, smokers, or coffee drinkers. In order for maximum human growth to occur, all symptoms of intrapsychic addiction must be dealt with (but perhaps not all at once).

## ALCOHOLISM/DRUG ADDICTION

The term alcoholism is used to describe addiction to alcohol. This is the most common of all addictions, the best researched and best understood. However, rarely in an adolescent is alcohol the only chemical used. The same problem in reverse applies to the term drug addiction. Most drug addicts will also use alcohol and many mistakenly believe that even though they are addicted to drugs, they can safely use alcohol.

The most encompassing of the terms described above is intra-psychic addiction, which is the substrate for a variety of addictive manifestations. Everyone who is chemically dependent is also in-trapsychically addicted. All alcoholics and drug addicts are chemically dependent, therefore, these terms are the narrowest in scope. Much of the literature which will be reviewed will refer to research in the alcoholism or drug addiction fields, simply because this is where the work has been done. Where possible, it will also be applied to the broader concept of intrapsychic addiction. Several groupings of childhood factors will now be discussed as they relate to the development of addiction.

## PHYSICAL FACTORS

A great deal of research has been done recently in an attempt to show that alcoholism is hereditary. Twin studies, genetic marker studies and adoption studies have been cited (Goodwin, 1978) as demonstrating that there is a clear predisposition to alcoholism in the children of alcoholic parents. The most recent estimate is that children of alcoholic parents are four times as likely to become alcoholic as children of nonalcoholic parents (Mendelson and Mello 1979). Similar studies are generally not available relating to dependency on other drugs. Descriptive studies of children born with physical withdrawal symptoms and with fetal alcohol effects have been reported (Jackson, 1981). It is not yet known whether the severity of the physical involvement positively correlates with the onset of chemical dependency.

These studies are important, however, in that living with parental alcoholism has been identified as a major risk factor. Children of alcoholic parents must be educated that if they choose to drink, they must drink cautiously. They must be alerted to the earliest possible signs of alcoholism. Of course the most conservative course for the child of an alcoholic is to abstain completely from alcohol.

Perhaps just as important a question to ask is "What do the nonal-coholic children of alcoholic parents look like?" Wegscheider and Wegscheider (1978) have described many of the roles which children of alcoholics assume: caretaker, problem child, forgotten child, and family pet. The mere fact that these roles are prominent indicates that intrapsychic addiction is present in the nonalcoholic children of alcoholic parents as well. In most cases where there is intrapsychic addiction, it is behaviorally manifested in some form or other. Therefore, if children of alcoholic parents do not become alcoholic, their addiction instead may be manifest in compulsive work, overeating, depression, chronically symptomatic physical illness, or some other symptom.

## PSYCHOLOGICAL FACTORS

When the term "psychological" is used here, it does not refer to diagnostic categories or classifications. This section is concerned with what happens in a child's formative years which contributes to the development of intrapsychic addiction. Again, it is this author's contention that all chemically dependent persons have intrapsychic addiction and that after detoxification is completed, most chemical dependency treatment relates to intrapsychic addiction.

Traditionally the age of seven or eight has been considered the age when a child reaches the "age of reason." The concept of the "age of reason" is generally not clearly understood by parents or educators, but there is a vague understanding that the child should be able to know the difference between right and wrong. Viewing reasoning solely as the ability to distinguish between right and wrong limits thinking to a moralistic framework. It would be more accurate to view reasoning as the ability to distinguish between what is healthy or unhealthy for the person in the holistic sense, that is, spiritually, emotionally, mentally, and physically.

The ability to reason implies several things. First, the person (in this case the child) must be exposed to a set of information to be used in the reasoning process. This information can come in the form of facts and data directed toward the intellect (e.g., parents discussing the pros and cons of drinking alcohol or taking drugs with their children or answering their child's questions on this topic). Information also comes to a person from the experiences of day to day living. These experiences can be translated into cognitive awareness as in the case of a child first tasting alcohol saying: "YUK! That tastes awful!" (personal experience) or a child observing an alcoholic laying on the sidewalk and commenting on the observation (vicarious experience). Experience can also result in subconscious knowledge that is repressed (e.g., my daddy told me that drinking was bad for people, but he drinks and sometimes gets drunk and is mean to me. Maybe I'm to blame for his getting drunk). Experiential knowledge is often more powerful and lasting, be it positive or negative, than intellectual knowledge in its impact on our ability to reason. Essentially, as far as the role of information in reasoning is concerned, if a child is not exposed to a given set of data (e.g., has no exposure at all to alcohol), that data will not be able to be used by the child in the reasoning process.

The second necessary ingredient in the reasoning process is that the child possess some measure of values and principles. Values and principles are learned from parents, older siblings and others with whom the child closely interacts. A value is something that is considered precious or rated highly by the one doing the valuing. A value, then, is something that we hold dear to us. For some people this might be an education or a good paying job. Others value relationships with other human beings, their Higher Power, and with themselves. Many people today do not have a healthy set of personal values because they do not own a set of principles upon which to hang their values. A principle is any generalization that provides a basis for reasoning or a guide for conduct or procedure. The Ten Commandments are examples of principles or guidelines by which a person can live. Both values and principles must be internalized by a child for the child to be able to reason.

Initially, children live by the values and principles imparted to them by their parents. Many children carry their parents' values and principles into adolescence and adulthood without challenging them except perhaps during periods of normal adolescent rebellion. The development of the ability to reason requires that the person examine his/her values and principles and make an independent choice about which to keep, let go or replace. Unfortunately, children today are exposed to values and principles based upon satisfaction of external desires: the necessity of having a beautiful body, a new car, a suburban home, and all the other pleasures the world has to offer. Some children are unhappy because they don't have what they feel the world owes them. Those who generally get everything discover that happiness does not come from satisfying external desires. Children with these types of values and principles do not have the grounding to make healthy personal choices and are therefore excellent candidates for addiction.

The final element which must be present for a person to be able to reason is a healthy concept of self. A great deal of popular literature has been written on this topic lately. This is a testimony to the pervasiveness of poor self-concept in our society. Poor self-concept is externally manifested by either too low an opinion of oneself or too great an opinion of oneself. It is important to understand that both are symptoms of the same problem: a lack of self-acceptance.

A person who is not in touch with his or her own value as a precious human being will be unable to say "no" consistently when confronted with unhealthy choices and will succumb to the need to please another rather than be true to self. This includes, of course, the choice which young people are forced to make today about drinking or taking drugs. When a child does not know his or her own value there are two factors which become predominant in the child's life: pain and fear. Both factors operate mostly subconsciously. The pain is intrapsychic and is felt as a lack of wholeness or a disconnectedness with oneself. The fear is of not measuring up or never being quite good enough, and therefore having to prove to oneself and everyone else again and again that one is worthwhile. It must be understood that this pain and fear are constantly present and color everything which the child does. The child never develops or loses the ability to express feelings and emotions naturally. Along with this goes the inability to accept responsibility for mistakes and to be honest with oneself. The child begins a pattern of reacting defensively in order to protect the fragile, frightened person within.

If a child is exposed to appropriate input from the environment, is given and accepts solid values and principles, and develops a healthy self concept, the ability to reason will follow. It must be noted that in the above discussion no mention was made of traumatic events as leading to an inability to reason with self. All too frequently today children are exposed to physical abuse, incest, parental discord, and other obviously emotionally disturbing events. It is easy to see how the ability to reason with self would be affected by these factors. However, lapses in the development of the ability to reason even without having obvious emotional trauma are more normal than abnormal in our society. It is not just a case of "bad parents" leading to addiction. So many parents who want to be loving and supportive toward their children are simply not able to teach their children to reason. The parents are as much victims as are their children after them. It is simply a fact that you can't pass on something that you don't have for yourself.

The ability to "reason with self" must be distinguished from the general "ability to reason" which most of us possess. Parents reading this article might think to themselves: my child is able to reason. He is bright in school and has decided that he wants to go to college one day. He is active in sports and is able to make split-second decisions on the basketball court. Reasoning in this sense is a function of intellectual and physical development. There are many people who have very well-developed intellectual reasoning abilities but very poor abilities to reason with self, which is a function of spiritual and emotional development. Essentially, reasoning with self is the ability to decide what is healthy for oneself at any given moment and then to accept responsibility for the consequences of that decision.

Books have been written about parenting and any attempt to explore all the facets of this subject is beyond the scope of this paper. However, several factors will be listed as being especially important to the development of the ability to reason with self.

- Physical Contact—copious doses of hugs and kisses
- Discipline—(as opposed to punishment)—setting limits and sticking to them—letting children know what consequence is attached to violation of these limits and following through
- Consistency—Don't say "no" to a child's request unless you mean "no." If you mean "no," don't allow yourself to be talked out of, begged, badgered or cajoled out of your decision.
- Share Yourself—Let your children know not only by what you say but also by what you do what your values and principles are.
- Share Feelings—Don't hide negative or positive feelings from your children. Let them know you are human.
- Educate Them—Talk with them about alcohol, drugs, sex, eating, gambling and all the other pleasures which can so easily become addictions.
- Share Your Spiritual Beliefs—Whatever your concept to a Higher Power is, talk with your children about it. Don't be afraid to let them see you acknowledge your belief in a God more powerful than you who is very real in your life.

## SOCIAL FACTORS

Childhood and adolescence are times of trial and error and experimentation. Even among children who are able to reason with self, there is a great deal of testing of oneself vis-à-vis others to see how they measure up and compare. This is a natural part of learning about oneself. The child who is able to reason with self is in possession of values and principles, information, and a healthy sense of self with which to compare the messages received from other children and the environment. Peer pressure is discussed as an important factor in the onset of adolescent alcohol and drug use. Certainly adolescence is a time of increased personal uncertainty and, therefore, vulnerability to outside forces. One of the dilemmas faced by adolescents is whether to accept the values and principles of others or to keep one's own. Adolescents who have been taught the ability to reason with self will generally choose to return to acceptance of the values and principles they have held previously. It must be stated that in spite of the best parental upbringing, free will means that children may choose to live by a different set of values and principles and may, therefore, end up addicted. This is a risk all parents take by simply choosing to be parents. It is generally true, however, that the basic relationship which must be developed is that with oneself. Relationships with others generally fall into place when our relationship with self is healthy.

## CONCLUSION

The model of addiction shown in Figure 1 will, hopefully, put into perspective much of the research that has sought to investigate the etiology of chemical dependency and the effectiveness of approaches to its treatment. Numerous causal factors have been examined including heredity, biochemical differences, sociocultural factors, association with emotional problems, and personality. In proposing this model it is suggested that the field look beyond these variables to the more fundamental factor of the person himself. Once the person has been established as the prime factor to be considered in the development of addiction, the contribution of the factors mentioned above can be put into proper perspective.

Evaluation research will then be able to look beyond abstinence, employment, physical improvement, family improvement and self-help program involvement as outcome variables. Changes within the person will also be studied as growth occurs in response to treatment.

# FIGURE 1.

## MODEL OF ADDICTION

From the preceding discussion, a model of addiction can be developed.

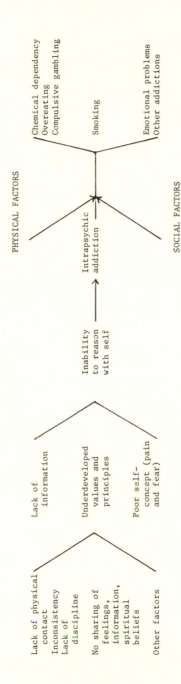

# REFERENCES

*Alcoholics Anonymous,* New York City: A. A. World Services Inc., 1976.

Culver, C. M., and Gert, B. *Philosophy in Medicine.* New York: Oxford University Press, 1981, 188-201.

Goodwin, D. "Alcohol and Heredity," *Arch. Gen. Psychiatry,* 1979, *36,* 57-61.

Jackson, G. W. "Fetal Alcohol Syndrome/Fetal Alcohol Effects: A Review," *Substance Abuse,* 1981-82, *3*(1), 3-8.

Love, M. C. Unpublished manuscript. Addiction Research, Inc. Deerfield Beach Fla., 1978.

Mendelson, J. H., and Mello, N. K. (Eds.). *The Diagnosis and Treatment of Alcoholism.* New York: McGraw-Hill, 1979.

Mule', S. J. (Ed.) *Behavior in Excess: An Examination of Volitional Disorders.* New York: Free Press, 1981.

Wegscheider, D., and Wegscheider, S. *Family Illness: Chemical Dependency.* Crystal, Minn., Nurturing Works, 1978.

# Influences on Adolescent Problem Behavior: Causes, Connections, and Contexts

Ardyth Norem-Hebeisen
Diane P. Hedin

**ABSTRACT.** This article examines the conceptual and empirical evidence for correlates of problem behavior in general and drug abuse in particular and develops a model for analyzing factors in drug abuse which may be useful in developing specific prevention programs to address the needs of adolescents.

Normal, healthy adolescent behavior can often be surprising or disturbing to parents and other adults. In recent years, however, powerful social factors have combined to produce a range of problem behavior among youth that is a source of even greater concern. The epidemic of youthful drug and alcohol abuse that began in the 1960s and continues into the present is an especially alarming manifestation of this trend.

The basic premise of this article is that peer influence can be an effective means of preventing drug abuse. Peer-group strategies are certainly not the only effective approach to drug abuse prevention, however, and peer influence is not the only factor associated with drug problems among youth. By stepping back and viewing the wider context of adolescent drug abuse and other problem behavior

This article is reprinted with minor revisions from *Adolescent Peer Pressure: Theory, Correlates, and Program Implications for Drug Abuse Prevention.* Washington, D.C.: National Institute on Drug Abuse, U. S. Department of Health and Human Services (Pub. No. (ADM) 81-1152), 1981, Pp. 21-46.

Ardyth Norem-Hebeisen is an assistant professor in social, psychological, and philosophical foundations of education in the College of Education, University of Minnesota. She is the author of *Peer Program for Youth* and a co-author of *Extend,* both of which deal with peer programs and are published by Augsburg Publishing Co., Minneapolis. Diane P. Hedin is assistant director of the Center for Youth Development and Research at the University of Minnesota. She conducts and publishes a poll of Minnesota youth on issues such as health, friendship, and drug use, and she conducted the first national study of school-based youth participation programs.

we can find clues to those issues that may be most important to address through peer-group strategies and programs. Without a broader view we are likely to oversimplify or misunderstand the role of peer influence in relation to other factors—and possibly, as a consequence, to build prevention programs on a weak theoretical foundation.

## SUBSTANCE ABUSE AS A PROBLEM BEHAVIOR

Not all alcohol and drug use is clearly problem behavior. In fact, if deviant or problem behavior is behavior that a considerable number of people view as reprehensible and beyond tolerance, then a large portion of experimental and occasional use cannot truly be viewed as deviant. For many youth experimentation with alcohol and drugs represents a push toward independence and adulthood (Mitchell, 1975). While one may criticize a society that has so few constructive rites of passage to adulthood that adolescents must use smoking, drinking, and getting high to mark the transition, these behaviors *in moderation* do not appear to be always problematic. Several studies show that while the majority use substances occasionally, only a minority become intensively involved (NIDA/ Jessor, 1978; NIDA/Johnston et al., 1979). Yet the more involved minority represents a significant proportion of youth, and the impairment and loss associated with their alcohol and drug use is of considerable consequence.

A number of studies indicate that drug and alcohol use among youth ranges from apparently normal behavior to obviously dysfunctional behavior accompanied by a wide variety of other behavioral and psychological difficulties. Dysfunctional use tends to be characterized by increasing quantity and the use of increasing varieties of both legal and illegal substances. It is often characterized by onset at an earlier age, and it tends to be associated with other kinds of dysfunctional behavior as well (Hamburg et al., 1974; NIDA/ Johnson et al., 1979; NIAAA, 1978).

### Overlapping Patterns of Problem Behavior

Alcohol and drug use are common among youth who also manifest other forms of dysfunctional behavior. Such youth are deviant in the sense that they participate in activities that are not a part of the mainstream of youth activities—activities that are considered to be contrary to social norms and consensually defined constructive behavior. Dropping out of school, truancy, running away from home, theft, teenage pregnancy, and mental health problems are examples of such problem behavior. The social costs of these behaviors are high for the individuals involved and for society as a whole.

Although today experimental drug use in the peer-group setting is often regarded as normal, not problematic; as young people use increasing quantities or varieties of both legal and illegal substances, experimental use can quickly become abuse. According to a 1978 national survey of drug use among high school seniors (NIDA/Johnston et al., 1979), by twelfth grade only about 10 percent of youth have never used any substance. About 90 percent have used alcoholic beverages once or more in the past twelve months; 65 percent have used them six or more times; and about 20 percent have used them weekly or more often. About 30 percent of young people report using cigarettes, 50 to 60 percent report using marijuana, and 20 percent report using other substances such as hallucinogens, sedatives, stimulants, tranquilizers, and opiates (polydrug use). A significant minority of youth are regular polydrug users. For each substance, youth report varying degrees of use, but there are clear patterns of overlapping use. For example, almost all marijuana users also use alcohol. Most youth who try or use other drugs also use alcohol and marijuana. There are some exceptions to these patterns. A few (but very few) young people report tobacco use but no alcohol use; a few smoke marijuana but do not drink alcoholic beverages.

Other problem behaviors often coincide with heavy drug use. Young people who drop out of school are also commonly found in the polydrug use category; only a few of them report no use (NIDA/Johnston et al., 1979). Youth who engage in theft or run away from home tend to be among those who drop out and among those who show some substance use. The more aberrant behaviors are likely to cluster in groups and to be characterized by more intense use of alcohol and a variety of drugs. This clustering of problem behaviors is a relatively recent social phenomenon—one that has been a source of great concern to parents, educators, policy makers, and other adults. (Additional research-based documentation of these patterns is cited in the "Behavior" section of the appendix to this article. The appendix summarizes the body of research on which the discussion in the following pages is based. This research is extensive and growing, so it was impossible in this relatively brief discussion to examine all the possible intercorrelations of problem behaviors and related factors. Instead, the research reviewed for this article constitutes a solid basis for discussing selected factors.)

## Correlates of Adolescent Problem Behavior

During the 1970s, when drug abuse and other forms of adolescent problem behavior were beginning to be viewed as symptoms of a deeper crisis among the nation's youth, a number of investigators tried to clarify our understanding of the factors leading both to initial and excessive use of substances among youth and to adolescent problem behavior generally. They also studied the processes by which people move into dysfunctional patterns of drug use and factors that appear to be important for the prevention and treatment of drug problems.

The literature based on these studies—commonly referred to as *correlate research*—is so vast that only a portion of it could be reviewed for this article. Although caution should be used in drawing sweeping conclusions from a review of studies based on such a wide range of data and methods, it is possible to examine this literature as a whole and find in it continuity and coherence. Despite the use of different measures, different populations, and different study methods in the studies that were reviewed, certain results recur consistently.

Since such a wide variety of correlates has been identified, we have organized them according to a systems model, which essentially creates separate categories of correlates and attempts to examine how the different categories relate to each other. We will discuss five categories that define an individual's relationship with self and environment: physical/genetic, cognitive/emotional, behavioral, social network, and societal/cultural.

*Physical/genetic* includes physical processes and functions. When we discuss alcohol and drug use, this category could include correlates such as hyperactivity, allergic reactions, heredity, and blood sugar level. Physical/genetic correlates such as early physical maturation may also be important when we consider aspects of school performance, delinquency, truancy, running away, sexual acting out, and other dysfunctional behavior.

*Cognitive/emotional* includes a wide variety of correlates such as the development of values, motivation, thought processes, and emotional processes. Research that considers other patterns of dysfunctional behavior may also focus on strategies used in problem solving, attribution of meaning, or dealing with depression or anxiety.

*Behavioral* correlates consist of those actions that others can observe an individual performing. In relation to dysfunctional behavior, these include acting out, manifest skill in problem solving, self-control, management of demanding tasks, communication skills, and task achievement of many kinds.

*Social network* correlates refer to that matrix of relationships in which each individual is enmeshed; they comprise that individual's social reality. They include peers, who have an influence on alcohol and drug use as well as on other behaviors; parents, who serve as models of drug use, ability to cope with stress, and social relationships (models that may be either complementary or contradictory to peer influence); teachers and students at school; fellow workers in a job setting; and people contacted through participation in extracurricular and religious activities.

*Societal/cultural* correlates are those influences that society and culture as a whole place on members of society. They include cultural expectations of youth; the influence of the mass media; and national and regional opinions about youth development, employment opportunities, drug and alcohol laws, truancy, vandalism, theft, sexual activity, and related behaviors.

As is evident from the accumulated body of correlate research summarized in the appendix, there are many similarities among youth who engage in various forms of problem behavior. Furthermore, many of the correlates associated with problem behavior—impulsiveness, irresponsibility, and rebelliousness, for example—are similar to each other. These similarities are most apparent in the cognitive/emotional, behavioral, and social network categories, as highlighted below:

— Cognitive/emotional correlates significantly related to a variety of problem behaviors include low self-esteem, impulsiveness, negative attitudes toward school, low cognitive development, and low academic aspirations.
— Behavioral correlates most frequently associated with other problem behaviors are school discipline problems, delinquent behavior, all types of antisocial behavior, and frequent use of cigarettes, alcohol, and other drugs. (In short, many types of problem behavior are closely correlated with each other.)

— Social network correlates most strongly associated with involvement in problem behavior include a variety of forms of family disorganization, inadequate parenting, poor parent-child relationships, and peer models.

Peer models for and approval of problem behavior are critically important social network correlates. They are almost always a part of the experience of those involved in drug and alcohol use, running away, adolescent pregnancy, premarital sex, and dropping out of school.

## Variables Affecting the Onset of Problem Behavior

How can we know when factors that are associated with problem behavior might actually lead to problem behavior? In a pure cause-and-effect sense, this is difficult to determine. If we could define precise causal relationships for such problem behaviors as drug abuse, drug abuse prevention would be a simple matter of applying scientifically exact technologies. It is, however, a much more complex and human process, and at present we can only speculate about the causes.

The growing body of research into drug abuse correlates does suggest some consistent patterns, however, and there is beginning to be a consensus among prevention theorists that can help us to understand, predict, and prevent problem behavior among adolescents (Robins et al., 1977; Robins, 1978). Problem behavior among youth almost always appears to be associated with a broader set of variables that subsume the correlates of problem behavior summarized above. The three variables that seem to occur most consistently in relation to problem behavior are stress, skill deficiencies, and situational constraints.

*Stress.* Youth experience stress in a variety of forms—for example, loss (of a parent or friend), rejection, abuse (sexual or physical), and failure in varying degrees of severity and across different aspects of their experience. At-risk youth are highly stressed; although all youth inevitably experience some stress, those with lower levels of stress appear to be less inclined toward problem behavior.

*Skill deficiencies.* Young people vary according to the kinds of skills they have for coping successfully with stress when it occurs. Important developmental skills relate to such tasks and life events as problem solving, communication, accurate self-assessment, and constructive processes for interpreting and understanding experiences. At-risk youth are often characterized by low attainment of such skills. Some youth who have adequate life-coping skills can deal effectively with high degrees of stress; others who lack such skills are more vulnerable.

*Situational constraints.* At the situational level the influence of the peer group is particularly important. Many teenagers' peers or role models encourage experimentation with high-risk behaviors such as substance abuse, precocious sexual activity, and vandalism. At-risk youth often find themselves in situations where problem behavior is expected and supported.

All of these variables can interact with each other, and they can contribute separately or collectively to the development of problem behavior. Figure 1 illustrates the nature of the possible interactions by presenting examples of the correlates of problem behavior from the appendix. As Figure 1 indicates, many correlates and variables can work together to determine whether or not a young person will become involved in substance abuse or other forms of problem behavior. The influences vary from individual to individual. No one factor by itself is either necessary or sufficient to produce problem behavior. Rather, it appears that the combination of varieties and degrees of factors produces a range of problem behavior of varying severity.

## A "COMMON COLD" METAPHOR

The conceptual approach described above can be seen in terms of a health problem that, although less serious, has been just as difficult to eradicate as drug abuse: the common cold.

To prevent a cold we have to pay attention to a wide variety of conditions that can be seen as corresponding to the three variables of stress, skill deficiency, and situational constraints. We try to maintain a proper balance of conditions in order to reduce our vulnerability, i.e., we try to reduce stress. Therefore, we try to maintain proper nutrition and get enough rest, fresh air, and exercise. To minimize exposure to pathogens, we stay away from people who are already sick with colds and we avoid extreme temperatures, i.e., we try to minimize situational constraints. Some of these efforts help us maintain a condition of balanced health, i.e., improve our coping

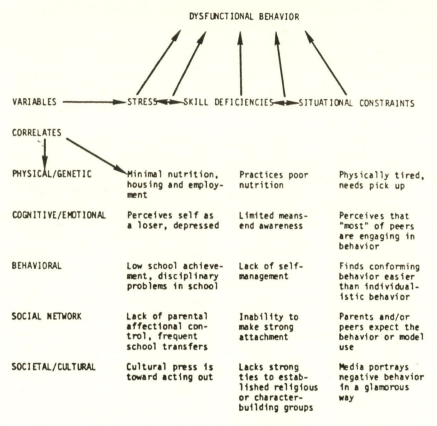

Figure 1

EXAMPLES OF FACTORS THAT INFLUENCE YOUTH TOWARD DYSFUNCTIONAL BEHAVIOR

DYSFUNCTIONAL BEHAVIOR

| VARIABLES | STRESS | SKILL DEFICIENCIES | SITUATIONAL CONSTRAINTS |
|---|---|---|---|
| CORRELATES | | | |
| PHYSICAL/GENETIC | Minimal nutrition, housing and employ-ment | Practices poor nutrition | Physically tired, needs pick up |
| COGNITIVE/EMOTIONAL | Perceives self as a loser, depressed | Limited means-end awareness | Perceives that "most" of peers are engaging in behavior |
| BEHAVIORAL | Low school achieve-ment, disciplinary problems in school | Lack of self-management | Finds conforming behavior easier than individual-istic behavior |
| SOCIAL NETWORK | Lack of parental affectional con-trol, frequent school transfers | Inability to make strong attachment | Parents and/or peers expect the behavior or model use |
| SOCIETAL/CULTURAL | Cultural press is toward acting out | Lacks strong ties to estab-lished religious or character-building groups | Media portrays negative behavior in a glamorous way |

skills, and others keep us from exposure to conditions that are known to contribute to physical breakdown when the body is vulnerable.

In a similar way, if we are to prevent alcohol and drug abuse and other problem behavior among youth, we need to maintain healthy, balanced conditions and reduce exposure to harmful influences. We must attempt to decrease physical and emotional stress and increase a wide range of coping skills. We must also create and maintain healthy, constructive environments and social situations. By max-imizing the survival, maintenance, and healthy growth of in-dividuals and groups, we can reduce the likelihood of problem behavior.

Yet other measures need to be taken to deal with the sometimes unavoidable circumstances that induce problems. An individual who has been raised to be mentally and physically sound and to cope successfully with stress may suddenly encounter extreme uncertainty, distress, or danger. If, at the same time, drugs and alcohol are readily available and there is strong social support for their use, the likelihood of use will increase (this happened to young soldiers in the Vietnam war). For adolescents, the influence of the drug-oriented peer culture can provide a similar jolt.

## RELATIONSHIP OF PEER INFLUENCE TO OTHER FACTORS AND IMPLICATIONS FOR PREVENTIONS PROGRAMMING

Given all the previously discussed factors that influence an adolescent's drug and alcohol use and related problem behavior (the five categories of correlates and the three major variables described above), where can a prevention program begin? Although a number of correlates are associated with problem behavior, one that appears frequently and exerts an undeniable influence is association with peers who also accept and exhibit such behavior. Peer influence certainly is not the only factor, or even in many cases the critical factor. Nevertheless, the growing importance of peer influence in normal, healthy adolescent development should alert us to the need for particular attention to peer influence in any discussion of problem behavior among adolescents.

The almost universal presence of peer-group conformity can be understood from several perspectives. Developmentally, adolescents derive progressively less protection and information from their parents, while at the same time they are receiving increasing support from and choosing more interaction with peers. For example, Clark et al. (1975) document a shift toward friends as an information source about drugs from seventh grade on. Utech and Hoving (1969) and Curtis (1974) find that parents decrease as reference sources as children grow older. While both report decreases in conformity to parents, only Utech and Hoving report increasing conformity to peers. Curtis indicates that respect for the advice and directions given by friends did not increase.

This difference in findings may be clarified in several ways. First, youth are not influenced equally by peers in all areas of life. Teenagers most strongly influence each other regarding dress and appearance, choice of leisure-time activities, language, and use of alcohol and drugs (Hedin and Simon, 1980). Parental influence is strongest with regard to moral and social values, vocational choice, and educational plans (Cooper et al., 1977). Further Stone et al. (1979) point out that some youth are more parent-oriented while others are more peer-oriented, and that choices with respect to drug use may differ according to those orientations. Indeed Jessor and Jessor (1977), Kandel (1978, 1975), and Lassey and Carolson (1980) have all documented that the degree of emotional closeness between parents and their adolescent children is a factor in drug use. Values consensus between parents and youth has also been noted by Jessor and Jessor (1977). For example, youth who are alienated from their parents who oppose use and who are at the same time friends with peers who favor use are more likely to use drugs and alcohol (Jessor and Jessor, 1977); Kandel, 1975; Edelbrock, 1980). The studies suggest that youth are more at risk if people in their dominant reference group use substances and less at risk if the group is comprised of nonusers. Peer-oriented youth are more at risk if their *friends* use substances; parent-oriented youth are more at risk if their *parents* are users.

Although parental influence is more important for some young people than for others, peer influence is the dominant factor for many teenagers' entrance into problem behaviors. Since peer influence is so clearly part of the problem, it must also be part of the solution. Peers not only influence each other negatively by manipulation and coercion, but also positively by offering advice, support, and the opportunity to discuss conflicting points of view (Kiesler and Kiesler, 1969; Shute 1975). In the peer group, attitudes, values, parental behavior, the school, and society are discussed, judged, and mediated. As participants in these groups, teenagers are influenced by their desire to conform to both stated and unstated group expectations. The way in which peer influence impels youth toward or away from drug experimentation is complex—but undeniably important.

## Peer Approaches in Prevention

The foregoing discussion of problem behavior notwithstanding, strong peer interaction and influence is a normal, necessary, and healthy part of adolescent development (Erikson, 1968). This natural tendency to rely on peers provides an opportunity to channel that very force toward healthy behavior and the promotion of the survival, maintenance, and growth of the individual. Peer groups have outstanding potential as an effective method for preventing problem behavior because they can readily be tailored to deal with so many of the factors related to stress reduction, building coping skills, and modifying situational constraints outlined previously. For example, the following types of peer programs can help to address many different factors associated earlier in this chapter with adolescent problem behavior.

— *Positive peer influence* programs can help to channel peer pressure in positive directions; they can also help to develop and enhance self-esteem and problem-solving and decision-making skills.
— *Peer teaching* programs address the need not just for useful information and skills among youth, particularly in relation to academic success in school; they also provide participating youth with meaningful roles and real-world responsibilities at a time when youth are increasingly isolated from such roles and responsibilities in the prolonged adolescence characteristic of our culture.
— *Peer counseling/facilitating/helping* programs assist young people in solving problems and coping with some of the challenges with which they are inevitably confronted in modern society. Family problems and problems with friends and school are commonly dealt with in these kinds of programs.
— *Peer participation* programs can function as a link between the world of peers and the world of adults by providing peers with real-world tasks and responsibilities and adult guidance in accomplishing them.

In short, peer programs can address all the major variables—stress, skill deficiency, and situational constraints—that the foregoing discussion has identified as being closely related to problem behavior. The growing popularity of peer-group strategies in schools and youth-service programs across the country attests to the appeal of these approaches, and research evidence has also begun to support their effectiveness.[1]

---

[1] For a more detailed discussion of these four types of peer programs, including exemplary models and how to plan and complement peer programs, see *Adolescent Peer Pressure: Theory, Correlates and Program Implications for Drug Abuse Prevention,* Rockville, MD: National Institute on Drug Abuse, 1981.

## IN CONCLUSION

This article has analyzed a broad spectrum of factors related to adolescent problem behavior and has proposed a theoretical approach both to the development of problem behavior and to ways of preventing it. Although we still know very little about actual cause-and-effect relationships, a number of closely related sociocultural correlates of adolescent problem behavior have been identified by various studies, and many of these recur consistently in relation to overlapping patterns of problem behavior. The role of peer influence is only one of many factors, but, given its significance in normal, healthy adolescent development, it is critical.

By providing as many opportunities as possible for healthy development and by minimizing risks we can reduce young people's vulnerability to problem behavior. Since anything that severely obstructs the survival, maintenance, or growth of an individual may lead to negative outcomes, an effective approach to the prevention of problem behavior calls for many kinds of simultaneous efforts. Prevention should work to minimize avoidable stress, abuse, and loss in the lives of young people. It should provide a wide range of constructive coping skills—skills that can promote healthy social and emotional development and thus help in the management of unavoidable stresses. Further, prevention should reduce the impact of situational factors that encourage drug and alcohol abuse.

Peer group approaches show great promise in accomplishing many of these ends. Peer programs can help young people to become more competent, to make meaningful contributions to their peer groups and their communities and, most important, to gain experience in functioning as effective and concerned human beings.

## REFERENCES

Ahlgren, A., Norem-Hebeisen, A. A., Hochhauser, M., and Garvin, J. "Antecedents of Smoking Among Pre-adolescents." Unpublished paper, the authors, 1980.

Allen, V. L., Felman, R. S., and Devin-Sheehan, L. Research on children tutoring children: A critical review. *Review of Educational Research,* 46(3):35, 1976.

Bachman, J. G., O'Malley, P. M., and Johnston, J. *Adolescence to Adulthood: Change and Stability in the Lives of Young Men.* Ann Arbor, MI: Survey Research Center, 1978.

Banks, M. H., Bewley, B. R., Bland, J. M., Dean, J. R., and Pollard, V. Long-term study of smoking by secondary school children. *Archives of Disease in Childhood,* 53(1):12-19, 1978.

Barnes, G. E. Solvent abuse: A review. *International Journal of the Addictions,* 14(1):1-26, 1979.

Blum, R. H. *Horatio Alger's Children.* San Francisco: Jossey-Bass, 1972

Blum, R. H., Garfield, E. F., Johnstone, J. L., and Magistad, J. G. Drug education: Further results and recommendations. *Journal of Drug Issues,* 8(4):379-425, 1978.

Braucht, G. N., Brakarsh, D., Follingstad, D., and Berry, K. L. Deviant drug use in adolescence: A review of psychosocial correlates. *Psychological Bulletin,* 79(2):92-106, 1973.

Brennan, T. Mapping the diversity among runaways: A descriptive multivariate analysis of selected social psychological background conditions. *Journal of Family Issues,* 1(2): 189-209, 1980.

Bronfenbrenner, U. Is early intervention effective? *Day Care and Early Education,* 2(2): 1-25, 1974.

Chilman, C. "The educational-vocational aspirations and behaviors of unmarried and married undergraduates at Syracuse University." Unpublished paper, the author, 1963.

Clark, R. E., Kowitz, A., and Duckworth, D. The influence of information sources and grade level on the diffusion and adoption of marijuana. *Journal of Drug Issues,* Spring:177-188, 1975.

Clarke, J. W., and Levine, E. L. Marijuana use, social discontent and political alienation: A study of high school youth. *American Political Science Review,* 65(2):120-130, 1971.

Coddington, R. D. The significance of life events as etiologic factors in the diseases of children. *Journal of Psychosomatic Research,* 16(1):7-18, 1972.

Cognetta, P. V., and Sprinthall, N. A. Students as teachers: Role taking as a means of promoting psychological and ethical development during adolescence. In: Sprinthall, N. A. and Mosher, R. L., eds. *Value Development . . . As the Aim of Education.* Schenectady, NY: Character Research Press, 1978.

Conger, J. *Adolescence and Youth.* New York: Harper and Row, 1973.

Conrad, D. "The Differential Impact of Experiential Programs on Secondary School Students." Unpublished doctoral dissertation, University of Minnesota, 1980. 152 pp.

Cooper, D. M., Olson, D., and Fournier, D. Adolescent drug use related to family support, self-esteem, and school behavior. *Center Quarterly Focus,* Spring:121-134, 1977.

Curtis, R. L. Parents and peers: Serendipity in a study of shifting reference sources. *Social Forces,* 52(3):368-375, 1974.

Cvetkovich, G., and Grote, B. "Psychological Factors Associated with Adolescent Premarital Coitus." Paper presented at the National Institute of Child Health and Human Development, Bethesda, MD, May 1976.

Davis, A. K.; Shute, R. E.; and Weener, J. M. Positive peer influence: School-based prevention of drug and alcohol abuse. *Health Education,* 8(4):18-32, 1977.

Donovan, J. E., and Jessor, R. Adolescent problem drinking: Psychosocial correlates in a national sample study. *Journal of Studies on Alcohol,* 39(9):1506-1524, 1978.

Duncan, D. F. Life stress as a precursor to adolescent drug dependence. *International Journal of the Addictions,* 12(8):1047-1056, 1977.

Edelbrock, C. Running away from home: Incidence and correlates among children and youth referred for mental health services. *Journal of Family Issues,* 1(2):210-228, 1980.

Ehrmann, W. *Premarital Dating Behavior.* New York: Holt, Rinehart and Winston, 1959.

Erikson, E. *Identity, Youth, and Crisis.* New York: W. W. Norton and Co., 1968.

Galli, N., and Stone, D. B. Psychological status of student drug users. *Journal of Drug Education,* 5(4):327-333, 1975.

Gallup, G. *The Gallup Poll, Public Opinion 1972-1977.* Vol. 2. Wilmington, DE: Scholarly Resources, Inc., 1978.

Goodwin, D. W., Schulsinger, F., Hermansen, L., Guze, S. B., and Winokur, G. Alcohol problems in adoptees raised apart from alcohol biologic parents. *Archives of General Psychiatry,* 28(3):238-243, 1973.

Goodwin, F. K., and Bunney, W. E. A psychobiological approach to affective illness. *Psychiatric Annals,* 3(2):19-53, 1973.

Haagen, C. H. "Social and Psychological Characteristics Associated with the Use of Marijuana by College Men." Unpublished master's thesis, Wesleyan University, 1970. 187 pp.

Hamburg, B. A., Kraemer, H. D., and Jahnke, W. A hierarchy of drug use in adolescence:

Behavioral and attitudinal correlates of substantial drug use. *American Journal of Psychiatry,* 132(11): 1155-1163, 1974.

Hanneman, G. J., and McEwen, W. J. The use and abuse of drugs: An analysis of mass media content. In: Ostman, R. E., ed. *Communication Research and Drug Education.* BeverlyHills, CA: Sage Publications, 1976.

Harbin, H. T., and Maziar, H. M. The families of drug abusers: A literature review. *Family Process,* 14(3):411-431, 1975.

Harris, L. H. Middle-class high school dropouts: Incidence of physical abuse, incest, sexual assault, loss, symptomatic behaviors, and emotional disturbance. Unpublished doctoral dissertation, University of Minnesota, 1980. 138 pp.

Hebeisen, A. *Peer Program for Youth.* Minneapolis: Augsburg Publishing, 1972.

Hedin, D. P. Evaluating experiential learning. *Character,* 1(4):2-9, 1980.

Hedin, D., Arneson, J., Resnick, M., and Wolfe, H. *Minnesota Youth Poll: Youths' Views on National Service and the Military Draft.* Miscellaneous Report 158. St. Paul, MN: University of Minnesota Agricultural Experiment Station, 1980.

Hedin, D., and Simon, P. *Minnesota Youth Poll: Youths' Views on Leisure Time, Friendship and Youth Organizations.* Miscellaneous Report 160. St. Paul, MN: University of Minnesota Agricultural Experiment Station, 1980.

Hunt, L. G., Farley, E. C., and Hunt, R. G. Spread of drug use in population of youths. In: Beschner, G. M., and Friedman, A. S., eds. *Youth Drug Abuse: Problems, Issues and Treatment.* Lexington, MA: Lexington Books, 1979.

Hurd, P. D., Johnson, C. A., Pechacek, T., Bast, L. P., Jacobs, D. R., and Luepker, R. V. Prevention of cigarette smoking in seventh grade students. *Journal of Behavioral Medicine,* in press.

Jessor, R., and Jessor, S. L. Theory-testing in longitudinal research on marijuana use. In: Kandel, D., ed. *Longitudinal Research on Drug Use: Empirical Findings and Methodological Issues.* Washington, D.C.: Halstead-Wiley, 1978.

Jessor, R., Carman, R. S., and Grossman, P. H. Expectations of need satisfaction and drinking patterns of college students. *Quarterly Journal of Studies on Alcohol,* 29(1-A): 101-116, 1968.

Jessor, R., and Jessor, S. L. *Problem Behavior and Psychosocial Development: A Longitudinal Study of Youth.* New York: Academic Press, 1977.

Johnson, C. A., and Murray, D. M. Personal Communication, 1980.

Johnson, D. W. Group processes: Influences of student-student interaction on school outcomes. In: McMillan, J., ed. *The Social Psychology of School Learning.* New York: Academic Press, 1980.

Kandel, D. Inter and intragenerational influences on adolescent marijuana use. *Journal of Social Issues,* 30(2):107-135, 1974.

Kandel, D. Stages in adolescent involvement in drug use. *Science,* 190(4217):912-914, 1975.

Kandel, D. Adolescent marijuana use: Role of parents and peers. *Science,* 181(4104):1067-1070, 1973.

Kandel, D. B.; Kessler, R. C.; and Margulies, R. Antecedents of adolescent initiation into stages of drug use: A developmental analysis. In: Kandel, D., ed. *Longitudinal Research on Drug Use: Empirical Findings and Methodological Issues.* Washington, D.C.: Halstead-Wiley, 1978.

Kantner, J., and Zeknik, M. Sexual experience in young unmarried women in the United States. *Family Planning Perspectives,* 4(4):9-18, 1972.

Kaplan, H. B. Increase in self-rejection as an antecedent of deviant responses. *Journal of Youth and Adolescence,* 4(3):281-292, 1975.

Kiesler, C., and Kiesler, S. *Conformity.* Reading, MA: Addison-Wesley, 1969.

Kinsey, A. C., Pomeroy, W., Martin, C. E., and Gebbard, P. *Sexual Behavior in the Human Female.* Philadelphia: W. B. Saunders Co., 1953.

Kohlberg, L., LaCrosse, J., and Ricks, D. The predictability of adult mental health from childhood behavior. In: Wolman, B., ed. *Handbook of Child Psychopathology.* New York: McGraw-Hill, 1970.

Konopka, G. *Young Girls: A Portrait of Adolescence.* Englewood Cliffs, NJ: Prentice-Hall, 1975.

Lassey, M. L., and Carolson, J. E. Drinking among rural youth: The dynamics of parental and peer influence. *International Journal of the Addictions,* 15(1):61–75, 1980.

Linn, L. S. Social identification and the use of marijuana. *International Journal of the Addictions,* 6(1):79–107, 1971.

Miller, P., and Simon, W. Adolescent sexual behavior: Context and change. *Social Problems,* 22(1):58–76, 1974.

Milman, D. H., and Wen-Huey, S. Patterns of illicit drug use among secondary school students. *Journal of Pediatrics,* 83(2):314–320, 1973.

Mitchell, J. J. *The Adolescent Predicament.* Toronto: Holt, Rinehart and Winston of Canada, 1975.

Moore, K., and Caldwell, B. *Out of Wedlock Childbearing.* Washington, D.C.: Urban Institute, 1977.

Mosher, R. L. Theory and practice: A new E.R.A. *Theory Into Practice,* 16(2):81–88, 1977.

Mosher, R. L., and Sullivan, P. R. A curriculum in moral education for adolescents. *Journal of Moral Education,* 5(2):159-172, 1976.

National Commission on Resources for Youth. Youth counsels youth: An introduction to peer co-counseling. New York: the Commission, 1979.

National Institute on Alcohol Abuse and Alcoholism. *Alcohol and Drug Use Among Teenagers: A Questionnaire Study,* by Wechsler, H., and Thum, D. Proceedings of the Second Annual Alcoholism Conference. Rockville, MD: the Institute, 1972. pp. 33-46.

National Institute on Alcohol Abuse and Alcoholism. *Third Special Report to the U.S. Congress on Alcohol and Health from the Secretary of Health, Education and Welfare.* Rockville, MD: the Institute, June 1978.

National Institute on Drug Abuse. Predicting time of onset of marijuana use: A developmental study of high school youth, by Jessor, R. In: Lettieri, D. J., ed. *Predicting Adolescent Drug Use: A Review of the Issues, Methods, and Correlates.* DHEW Pub. No. (ADM)76-299. Washington, D.C.: Supt. of Docs., U.S. Govt. Print. Off., 1975a.

National Institute on Drug Abuse. Teenage drug use: A search for causes and consequences, by Smith, G. M. In: Lettieri, D. J., ed. *Predicting Adolescent Drug Use: A Review of the Issues, Methods, and Correlates.* DHEW Pub. No. (ADM)76-299. Washington, D.C.: Supt. of Docs., U.S. Govt. Print. off., 1975b.

National Institute on Drug Abuse. Some comments on the relationship of selected criteria variables to adolescent illicit drug use, by Kandel, D. In: Lettieri, D. J., ed. *Predicting Adolescent Drug Abuse: A Review of Issues, Methods, and Correlates.* DHEW Pub. No. (ADM)76-299. Washington, D.C.: Supt. of Docs., U.S. Govt. Print. Off., 1975c.

National Institute on Drug Abuse. A review of recent psychosocial research, by Jessor, R. In: DuPont, R. R., Goldstein, A., and O'Donnell, J. A., eds. *Handbook on Drug Abuse.* Washington, D.C.: Supt. of Docs., U.S. Govt. Print. off., 1978.

National Institute on Drug Abuse. *Drugs and the Class of '78: Behaviors, Attitudes and Recent National Trends,* by Johnston, L. D., Bachman, J. G., and O'Malley, P. M. DHEW Pub. No. (ADM) 79-877. Washington, D.C.: Supt. of Docs., U.S. Govt. Print. Off., 1979.

National Institute of Health. *Adolescent Sexuality in a Changing Society: Social and Psychological Perspectives,* by Chilman, C. DHEW Pub. No. (NIH)79-1426. Washington, D.C.: Supt. of Docs., U.S. Govt. Print. Off., 1979.

Norem-Hebeisen, A. A., and Martin, F. B. *Parental Support as an Approach to Primary Prevention of Chemical Abuse.* Final project report submitted to St. Paul Companies. St. Paul, MN: the Companies, 1980.

Nylander, I., and Rydelius, P. A. The relapse of drunkenness in non-asocial teenage boys. *Acta Psychiatrica Scandinavica,* 49(4):435–443, 1973.

O'Dowd, M. M. Family supportiveness related to illicit drug use immunity. Unpublished doctoral dissertation, University of Maryland, 1973, 131 pp.

Office of Education. *The Education of Adolescents: The Final Report and Recommendations of the National Panel on High School and Adolescent Education.* DHEW Pub. No. (OE)76–0004. Washington, D.C.: Supt. of Docs., U.S. Govt. Print. Off., 1976.

Office of Education. *Early School Leavers: Position Paper.* Washington, D.C.: Bureau of Occupational and Adult Education, 1978.

Paolitto, D. The effects of cross-age tutoring on adolescence: An inquiry into theoretical assumptions. *Review of Educational Research,* 44(2):241–257, 1976.

Paton, S., Kessler, R. C., and Kandel, D. Depressive mood and adolescent illicit drug use: A longitudinal analysis. *Journal of Genetic Psychology,* 131(2):267–289, 1977.

Perry, C., Killen, J., Telch, M., Linkard, L. A., and Danaher, B. G. Modifying smoking behavior of teenagers: A school-based intervention. *American Journal of Public Health,* 70(7):722–725, 1980.

President's Science Advisory Committee. *Youth: Transition to Adulthood,* by Coleman, J. S. Chicago: University of Chicago Press, 1974.

Robins, L. N. Sturdy childhood predictors of adult antisocial behavior; Replications from longitudinal studies. *Psychological Medicine,* 8(4):611–622, 1978.

Robins, L. N., Davis, D. H., and Wish, E. Detecting predictors of rare events: Demographic, family, and personal deviances as predictors of stages in progression toward narcotic addiction. In: Strauss, J. S., Babigian, H., and Ross, M. A. eds. *The Origins and Course of Psychopathology: Methods to Longitudinal Research.* New York: Plenum, 1977.

Schuckit, M. A., Goodwin, D. W., and Winkour, G. Study of alcoholism in half-siblings. *American Journal of Psychiatry,* 128(9):1132–1136, 1972.

Schulsinger, F. Biological psychopathology. *Annual Review of Psychology,* 31:583–606, 1980.

Shute, R. E. The impact of peer pressure on the verbally expressed drug attitudes of male college students. *American Journal of Drug and Alcohol Abuse,* 2(2):231–243, 1975.

Smart, R. T., and Gray, G. Parental and peer influences as correlates of problem drinking among high school students. *International Journal of the Addictions,* 14(7):905–917, 1979.

Smith, G. M., and Fogg, C. P. Psychological predictors of early use, late use, and nonuse of marijuana among teenage students. In: Kandel, D., ed. *Longitudinal Research on Drug Use: Empirical Findings and Methodological Issues.* Washington, D.C.: Halstead-Wiley, 1978.

Sorensen, R. *Adolescent Sexuality in Contemporary America.* New York: World Publishing Co., 1973.

Spivack, G., Platt, J. J., and Shure, M. B. *The Problem-Solving Approach to Adjustment.* San Francisco: Jossey-Bass, 1976.

Spyker, J. M. Assessing the impact of low level chemicals on development: behavioral and latent effects. *Pharmacology Society Symposium: Federation Proceedings,* 34(9):1835–1844, 1975.

Stone, L. H., Miranne, A. C., and Ellis, G. J. Parent-peer influence as a predictor of marijuana use. *Adolescence,* 14(53):113–122, 1979.

Utech, D. A., and Hoving, K. L. Parents and peers as competing influences in the decisions of children of differing ages. *Journal of Social Psychology,* 78(2):267-274, 1969.

Vener, A., and Stewart, C. Adolescent sexual behavior in middle America revisited: 1970-73. *Journal of Marriage and the Family,* 36(4):728–735, 1974.

Vesell, E. S. Introduction: Genetic and environment factors affecting drug response in man. *Pharmacology Society Symposium: Federation Proceedings,* 31(4):1253–1269, 1972.

# APPENDIX

This appendix summarizes the research on factors relating to alcohol and drug use, running away, premarital intercourse, adolescent pregnancy, dropping out of school, and mental health problems referred to throughout the article.

For a significant number of subjects, research findings point to events, influences, and personal characteristics that frequently appear to occur before the onset of problem behavior. These we call *antecedents*. Research also documents events, influences, and personal characteristics that tend to be present at the time individuals are engaging the problem behavior. These we call *concomitants*.

For those interested in the prevention of problem behavior during adolescence, the distinction can be useful. For example, if research has clearly demonstrated that a factor such as poor problem-solving skills is usually present prior to and while a person is experiencing dysfunction behavior, an intervention to enhance problem solving skills would be clearly indicated. However, if research showed that poor problem-solving skills were only a concomitant of the dysfunctional behavior, this factor probably would not be so important. (One might assume in such a case that the dysfunctional behavior led to a decline in problem-solving skills.) Consequently, although information about concomitants can suggest directions for prevention programming, it is not as cogent as information about antecedents. In order to provide the reader with a clearer picture of the various factors that contribute to dysfunctional behavior, the appendix is divided into two distinct categories: antecedents and concomitants. Some of the factors may be found listed in both categories. It should be noted, however, that such correlations are far from perfect; there are many exceptions whereby people with these characteristics are not drug abusers and vice versa.

## ANTECEDENTS

## CONCOMITANTS

### PHYSICAL/GENETIC

Failure to meet basic survival needs, health care, nutrition, housing, employment found prior to mental health problems (Bronfenbrenner, 1974)

Early maturing males, but not females, were sexually experienced at very young ages (Kinsey et al., 1953; Chilman, 1963)

Girls who become pregnant entered adolescence earlier than normal (Moore and Caldwell, 1977)

Genetic factors appear to play a role in the development of alcohol problems (Schuckits et al., 1972; Goodwin et al., 1973) and also in mental health problems and suicide (Schulsinger, 1980)

Genetic factors are associated with acute toxic reactions to drugs (Vesell, 1972)

Excessive use of marijuana may result in cardiovascular distress and injury (Johnson and Murray, 1980)

Individuals are more vulnerable to adverse effects of toxic substances on brain during childhood and adolescence (Spyker, 1975)

ANTECEDENTS                                    CONCOMITANTS

COGNITIVE/EMOTIONAL

Negative attitude toward school and low self-esteem found to precede onset of drug use (Ahlgren et al., 1980)

Low sense of psychological well being precedes onset of marijuana use (Smith and Fogg, 1978; Paton et al., 1977; Haagen, 1970)

Low self-esteem regarding school found prior to onset of drug use (Norem-Hebeisen, 1980; NIDA/Smith, 1975b)

High rebelliousness, untrustworthiness, sociability, and impulsive traits found in later drug users (NIDA/Smith, 1975b)

Lower ego maturity predicts psychopathology in adults (Kohlberg et al., 1970)

Scores of later premaritally pregnant girls were somewhat higher with respect to being more energetic, nonconformist, more outgoing, and socially active (Moore and Caldwell, 1977)

Tolerance of deviance strongly predicts alcohol and drug use, radical politics, delinquency, premarital sex (Jessor and Jessor, 1977)

Inconsistency between one's own and one's parents' opinions about drug use strongly predicts marijuana use (Jessor and Jessor, 1977)

Disagreement with parents' opinions about drinking predicts frequency of drunkenness (Jessor and Jessor, 1977)

Lower academic aspirations predict marijuana use (Jessor and Jessor, 1978)

Psychedelic drug use is associated with high scores on measures of alienation and search for meaning, dissillusionment and rebellion, need for stimulation, search for self-definition, seeking relief from anxiety and tension, high need for novelty, insecurity, egocentricism, shyness, feeling inadequate, depression, and tenseness (Braucht et al., 1973)

Dislike of school is associated with initial drug use (Ahlgren et al., 1980), dropping out of school (Bachman et al., 1978), running away from home (Brennan, 1980). Onset of marijuana use is associated with higher scores on political, personal, and family estrangement scales (Clarke and Levine, 1971)

Lower educational aspiration correlates with dropping out of school (Bachman et al., 1978), illicit drug use (Milman and Wen-Huey, 1973), and pregnancy (Chilman, 1963)

Less adequate problem solving is found among both drug users and youth with mental health problems (Spivack et al., 1976)

Lower expectation of getting one's needs met is more frequent among heavier drinkers (Jessor et al., 1968)

Lower commitment to traditional values is associated with premarital intercourse (Vener and Stewart, 1974)

Lower religiosity is associated with premarital intercourse (Jessor and Jessor, 1977; Cvetkovich and Grote, 1976) and drug use (Jessor and Jessor, 1977)

Problem drinking seems more associated with personality factors such as alienation, rather than parent and peer variables (Smart and Gray, 1979)

ANTECEDENTS                    CONCOMITANTS

COGNITIVE/EMOTIONAL (continued)

Lower cognitive development is associated with drug use (Spivack et al., 1976), premarital intercourse and pregnancy (NIH/Chilman, 1979)

Higher life stress scores are found in drug-dependent adolescents (Duncan, 1977) and those with mental health problems (Coddington, 1972)

Risk taking and sensation seeking is associated with premarital intercourse (Cvetkovich and Grote, 1976)

Lower self-esteem is associated with dropping out of school (Bachman et al., 1978), premarital intercourse (Cvetkovich and Grote, 1976), and running away (Brennan, 1980)

Concern about parents' drug use, and siblings' drug use, are correlated with dropping out of school (Harris, 1980)

Impulsive, fatalistic attitudes and lack of long-term goals are associated with dropping out of school (Conger 1973, Bachman et al., 1978)

BEHAVIORAL

Low school achievement predicts drug abuse (NIDA/Smith, 1975b; Jessor and Jessor, 1977), dropping out of school (Bachman et al., 1978), and mental health problems (Kohlberg et al., 1970)

Frequent cigarette smoking predicts drug use (Smith et al., 1975) and dropping out of school (Bachman et al., 1978)

Involvement in minor delinquent activities predicts drug use and dropping out of school (Bachman et al., 1978) and onset of use of hard liquor (NIDA/Kandel, 1975c)

Disciplinary problems in school predict drug use and dropping out of school (Bachman et al., 1978; Nylander and Rydelius, 1973)

Lack of success in attainment of school goals correlates with alcohol and marijuana use (Cooper et al., 1977), use of illicit drugs (Milman and Wen-Huey, 1973), promiscuity (Sorenson, 1973)

Frequency of school absenteeism correlates with increasing levels of drug use (Cooper et al., 1977) and dropping out of school (Office of Education, 1978)

Narcotic addicts have been found to be immature, insecure, irresponsible, egocentric, hedonistic, and lacking in personal controls (Braucht et al., 1973)

Frequent use of alcohol and drugs is associated with premarital intercourse (Vener and Stewart, 1974; Jessor and Jessor 1977) and running away from home (Edelbrock, 1980)

| ANTECEDENTS | CONCOMITANTS |
|---|---|

## BEHAVIORAL (continued)

Delinquent and deviant behavior predicts subsequent drug use (Jessor and Jessor, 1978; NIDA/Johnston, 1979, Kandel, 1973)

All types of antisocial behavior in childhood predict a high level of antisocial behavior in adulthood (Robins, 1978)

Heavy drug use and use of hard drugs is associated with promiscuity (Vener and Stewart, 1974)

Nonvirgin females and males are more likely to engage in delinquent behavior (Vener and Stewart, 1974)

## SOCIAL NETWORK

Parental use of hard liquor predicts use of marijuana by children and transition to other drugs (Kandel, 1974)

Parental divorce, arrest, and drug use problems predict liability to addiction (Robins et al., 1977)

Lack of closeness between parents and children predicts drug use (Kandel, 1974)

High level of adolescent peer activity predicts marijuana use (Kandel, 1974)

Pattern of drug use and problem behavior by close friends is a strong predictor of marijuana use (Kandel, 1974) and alcohol abuse (Jessor and Jessor, 1977)

Lack of an enduring relationship involving intensive interaction predicts mental health problems (Bronfenbrenner, 1974)

Stressful families and broken homes precede dropping out of school (Bachman et al., 1978)

Dropout-prone youth in a middle-class school had a high incidence of victimization (physical abuse, incest, or sexual assault) and loss (death of a family member or friend, moves, or school transfers) (Harris, 1980)

Family factors such as parental and sibling drug use, family disorganization, father unemployed, and one or both parents missing are associated with solvent abuse (Barnes, 1979)

Frequent drug use is associated with a perceived lack of parental support (Cooper et al., 1977; O'Dowd, 1973; Blum, 1972)

Male addicts lack identification with a positive male figure (Harbin and Maziar, 1975)

Greater heterosexual activity is associated with frequent drug use (Milman and Wen-Huey, 1973)

Family emphasis on independence instead of self-discipline and community responsibility is associated with frequent drug use (Blum et al., 1978)

Same-sex parents and siblings serve as "models" for smoking by adolescents (Banks et al., 1978)

Frequent drug users found to have less supportive perspective (O'Dowd, 1973)

Boys who were frequently drunk often had mentally ill or alcoholic fathers (Nylander and Rydelius, 1973)

Lack of consistent parental discipline is associated with premarital intercourse (Ehrmann, 1959; Cvetkovich and Grote, 1976)

ANTECEDENTS                          CONCOMITANTS

SOCIAL NETWORK (continued)

Nonvirgin females were more apt to be in one-parent families, in a variety of home situations (such as substitute parents), and in poor communication with parents (Kantner and Zelnick, 1972; NIH/Chilman, 1979; Sorenson, 1973)

High parental and peer acceptance of deviance, modeling and approving deviance by friends, and frequent conflict with parents were associated with premarital intercourse (Jessor and Jessor, 1977)

Nonvirgin females with many sexual partners ranked high on peer involvement and low on parent involvement (Miller and Simon, 1974)

Rejecting parents are associated with children who are frequent runaways (Edelbrock, 1980)

Poor relationships with parents, high family stress, and low educational attainment of parents is associated with dropping out of school (Office of Education 1978; Harris, 1980; Bachman et al., 1978)

Low-income, minority youth were more likely to be school dropouts (Bachman et al., 1978)

There is a strong association between poverty and premarital intercourse and pregnancy among black adolescent girls (Kantner and Zelnick, 1972)

SOCIETAL/CULTURAL

Adolescent drug use has grown as the broader society increasingly becomes a drug culture (Conger, 1973)

Growth of new drugs in high schools is sudden and sporadic—a form of fad behavior (Hunt et al., 1979)

Equal rights for women, a decrease in early marriages, and more permissive attitudes toward sexual behavior may be reasons for increased rates of premarital intercourse and adolescent pregnancy (NIH/Chilman, 1979)

ANTECEDENTS                    CONCOMITANTS

SOCIAL/CULTURAL (continued)

Portrayal of drugs as glamorous
stimulates drug use by youth (Hanneman
and McEwen, 1976)

# Reducing Black Adolescents' Drug Use: Family Revisited

Laura J. Lee

**ABSTRACT.** This article focuses on prevention and reduction of drug use among Black adolescents. The family is considered to be a major source in preparing children to handle adolescent stresses such as drug involvement pressures. Primary prevention of drug use begins in early childhood. The family is an underutilized and minimally acknowledged resource in drug abuse prevention efforts. The discussion centers on a review of research findings intimately related to adolescent drug use and Black family issues. An argument is made for a national family policy in support of all American families. Young families are a prime area for the investment of resources. Now and in the future, the American family represents the best primary prevention program available.

This paper focuses on the primary prevention and reduction of drug use by Black adolescents. The discussion is framed in the perspective that although there have been and are a multitude of approaches to primary prevention of drug abuse, the American family as a vehicle of prevention has been underutilized and minimally acknowledged. Families frequently are focused upon for the etiology of pathology, but rarely given top billing as an important ally in the struggle against drug abuse. The article reviews family related antecedents from research identified as contributing to the phenomenon of drug abuse by Blacks, draws implications from the antecedents and recommends directions for moving toward reducing and preventing drug abuse in conjunction with the family.

Generalizations about any segment of the population are difficult and risky. Each adolescent is a unique individual who is the sum total of his life experiences. Concurrently, he interacts with and is acted upon by social, economic and political forces in his environment, yet there are human needs and processes commonly accepted

Laura J. Lee is in the School of Social Work at the University of Pennsylvania, Philadelphia, PA 19104. Reprint requests should be addressed to the author.

*57*

and associated with adolescent years, roughly between the ages of 12-22 years. Certainly, a growth and development period precedes adolescence. It is during this period from infancy forward that the seeds of prevention can be planted and nurtured in hopes of preventing and minimizing adolescent problems, drug abuse included.

## THE CONCEPT OF DRUG ABUSE

The socially acceptable notion about drug abuse is that it needs to be prevented. "Drug abuse instead of referring to a topology of drug-using behaviors, has become a shorthand term society uses to differentiate between licit and illicit drug use" (NCMDA, 1973, p. 13). These two categories overlook the frequency with which a drug is used, method of administration, dosage and situations in which a drug is used (Goldberg and Meyers, 1980, p. 149). The National Commission on Marihuana and Drug Abuse identified five categories of drug using behavior, each having unique potential for the user's dysfunctioning and the potential purpose of preventive effort levels. These categories or levels of use are: experimental; recreational; circumstantial; intensive and compulsive. Preventive or interventive efforts must clearly identify goals and objectives in relation to a specific level of drug use. This paper is focused on prevention and reduction of intensive drug use by Black adolescents. Varied studies of addicts generally found that the onset of drug addiction for Blacks occurred between the ages of 14 and 19 years (Brotman and Freedman, 1968; Callan and Patterson, 1973; Chambers, 1974; Force, 1974; Gleaser, 1971; Halikas, 1976; Stephens, 1974). Prevention needs to occur many years before age 14.

Drug abuse is not a monolithic social problem. It is but one symptomatic cell in a web of interrelated dynamics and conditions that exist in our complex society. Minority groups tend to view substance abuse as a comprehensive social problem (National Institute on Drug Abuse, A Guide . . . 1981).

The concept of primary prevention of drug abuse has been around for several decades. It is a difficult concept to apply even though imminently logical. The human being is affected by an infinite number of conditions and experiences that cannot be controlled, even if it were desirable. In direct relation to the aging of our nation and culture, the wisdom and knowledge about human behavior expands and becomes more complex. Yet, some facts are known and change rather slowly. The industrialized United States is a drug oriented culture. Many persons' physical and emotional lives are wedded to licit and illicit drugs. Manatt (1982) warns that all children are growing up in an enviornment that exposes them to drugs and while parents are the child's main defense against these pressures, they are up against powerful social and economic forces. In terms of parental influence, Glynn (1981, p. 69) concluded that "the most effective family influences appear to be those that are developed in advance of adolescence. Satisfactory family relationships and climate, emotional support and moderation in the use of alcohol are influences that appear to delay or diminish adolescent initiation into drug use. These are influences that are developed over a long period of time and attempts to make up for their absence by measures such as sharp increases in parental control of the adolescents' behavior may lead to increased rather than diminished drug use."

Research into drug abuse correlates suggests some consistent patterns that may predict adolescent behavior such as drug abuse. "The three variables that seem to occur most consistently in relation to adolescent problem behavior are stress, skill deficiencies and situational constraints (Norem-Hebeisen and Hedin, 1981, p. 25).

## SELECTED FINDINGS

Part of prevention is knowing what is to be prevented. If intensive drug use by Black adolescents is to be prevented or reduced, data on the undesirable end product (the intensive adolescent and adult user of drugs) is useful in pinpointing contributors to the undesirable condition. Propositions have mainly been culled from drug abuse research studies that related to and/or included a representative or predominant sample of Black adolescents and adults. Black adolescent and family relatedness was the major criterion used in selecting findings. Reference to sex or socioeconomic status were not criteria. An undefined criterion was that the finding have the practical, concrete quality of being amendable to solution or modification.

## FAMILY LIFE ISSUES

Drug use was found to be lower among adolescents who had strong family ties (Globetti and Brigance, 1974). Family instability and lack of cohesiveness were more intense for drug users at an early age. The nuclear group made a difference between ages 6 years and 12 years. For older adolescent non-users, their families may have disintegrated during the teen years, but the earlier family experience seemed to sustain them (Craig and Brown, 1975). Lukoff and Brook (1974) directed attention toward the significance of disjunction between the family generations as a probability in an individual affiliating with drug users. The researchers posited that the decline in family legitimacy facilitated the intrusion of other socializing agents (mainly peer groups with divergent cultural content from the parent). These processes were viewed as antecedent to certain youngsters' experimenting with drugs.

A number of studies reenforced the finding that a large percentage of Black drug abusers are the product of broken or single parent homes (Craig and Brown, 1975; Waldorf, 1973; Vaillant, 1966; Chambers, 1970; Chambers et al., 1958; Chein, 1964). A Census Bureau study reported that twenty percent of all U.S. minors live with one parent and the divorce rate among Blacks went from 62 per 1000 in 1960 to 233 per 1000 in 1981 (Census Bureau, 1982). For Black children, the possibility of being reared by a single caregiver is increasing. In theory, total responsibility for parenting by a single person mandates periods of intense stress that may be diluted or shared if a second parent were present. Among Black drug abusers, a notable percentage had fathers who were absent. Robins (1967) noted that 56% of drug-using delinquents were without fathers during their teen years. Bates' study (1968) of 99 addicts in Lexington revealed 48.9% had not had the support of fathers. Goldsmith et al. (1972) investigated a sample of persons receiving methadone and found that 60% of the addicts had been reared in homes where the father was not present. One background factor with incarcerated addicts was the tendency to have been reared by dominant mothers who sheltered and overindulged them (Roebuck, 1962). Marital and family stability appear to influence drug use. Callan and Patterson (1973) associated unstable marital and family situations with a higher prevalence of drug use among young persons.

Varenhorst (1981) discussed the social and cultural development needs of adolescents. One such need is more help in developing social competence. This means learning how to cope and survive in a complex world with fewer opportunities to learn from an adult model. In a study of Black male adult addicts, Halikas (1976) found that 15% had some first degree family member with a drug problem and while children, 44% had admired some adult addict. Craig and Brown had similar findings from a Black adolescent population: thirty-two percent of the drug users reported members of their immediate families (usually siblings) and fourteen percent of their extended families as drug users. In this same study, two percent of the non-users reported drug use by members of their immediate family. These findings suggest a closer look at family members whose behavior teaches children through example. Intergenerational and extended family contacts are common for most Blacks. Family members serve as role models.

Continuing the theme of family members modeling behavior, Stenmark et al. (1974) explored the hypothesis that parents who used drugs (including alcohol) would be more likely to have adolescent children who used drugs than parents who did not use those substances, or who used them less frequently. For Blacks, parents' use of alcohol was consistently positively correlated with juvenile substance use. The investigators argued that efforts to alter the use of alcohol and other drugs by family adults is prerequisite to changes in drug use patterns among adolescents.

A particular Black family strength useful in preventing drug abuse is the evidence that Black drug users felt less alienated than white drug users from family, school and community. Black users and non-users of drugs resembled each other regarding family cohesiveness and tended to show greater family integrity than either white or Puerto Rican drug users (Chein, 1964; Nail et al., 1974). Historically, agencies and programs discriminated in the provision of services to Black persons who needed help. In the 60s expanded service opportunities and offerings were provided to Blacks. The present reality is that in general, informal social support continues to be provided by Black families. Taylor et al. (1982) found that family closeness and frequency of contact were positively associated with the frequency of support received. The family's economic resources influence the quality of life members are able to have. For Black families, employment is a critical issue.

## EMPLOYMENT

Since World War II, unemployment rates for Black youths have risen much more rapidly than for white youths. Today's continuing rate of unemployment among Black adolescents has been viewed by some persons as a direct contributor to drug abuse. "Normal" adolescents are young persons with high energy levels, striving toward adulthood and independence. For some, unable to have the status symbol and autonomy of employment, self-directed depression, frustration and anger replace the American dream. Without steady employment, it is impossible to progress on the socioeconomic ladder. Major trends in race differentials in youth employment and labor force participation since World War II have indicated a deterioration in the relative position of Black teenagers during the full postwar era; of Blacks in their twenties since 1970, and improvement since 1960 in the relative wages and occupational standing of young Blacks (Mare and Winship, 1980). Elimination of some unskilled jobs; the increasing tendency of Black youths to substitute schooling for work has reduced their labor market participation. Schools and the military screen-in those youths who would most likely be employed were they not in school or in service. Mare and Winship further concluded that as racial equality in other spheres has improved, differentials in the labor market have been revealed. "In the past, racial disparities in the youth labor market were concealed because many Black youths left school before whites and took jobs in the lowest-wage, lowest-skill sector of the economy. Now that jobs are scarce and Black youths match whites in schooling patterns, racial disparities are not revealed" (p. 34). These authors offer one description of the status of employment conditions for Black young persons. In a society where the work ethic provides a part of the individual's credibility and definition of self, lack of available employment is a major stress for Black adolescents. Helmer and Vietorisz (1974) reviewed the history of the U.S. labor market and the responsiveness of narcotic use. They concluded that concern about narcotics, and the intensity and focus of law enforcements have been functions of the condition of the labor market. Such response has provided at the same time a method for pitting the class against itself by identifying ethnic or racial minorities as scapegoats for larger and more fundamental social ills. Bates' (1968) survey of Black adult male addicts showed that a large number had never started a specific occupational career. Within the same sample, addicts who started steady work had extensive unemployment after starting drug use. The Glaser et al. (1971) study included the finding that addicts were more involved in illegitimate activities as youths and, as a result, less successful in education and employment, so turned to drug use as more gratifying behavior. For Blacks, especially youth, the stress of the dire employment situation renders an oppressed group even more vulnerable and erodes the integrity of the family unit. A family's economic condition and employment are interlocked with their place of residence.

## RESIDENTIAL COMMUNITY

In terms of socioeconomic status, Chein (1964) found that drug use among male adolescents was concentrated in those census tracts that constituted the most underprivileged, crowded and dilapidated areas of the city. Drug use was the highest where income and education were the lowest and when there was the greatest break-down in family life. Black drug users came from more deprived homes than Black non-users. The characteristic of urbanicity and drug abuse has been well documented. Black youths in cities have a higer probability of involvement with drugs. More concentrated law enforcement agencies, schools, residential proximity and availability and access to drugs are some of the better known reasons why the drug phenomenon is centralized in cities.

Researchers have easier access to youths in an urban and/or a contained geographic area. It could well be that rural Black adolescents are understudied, therefore the total study population is skewed in favor of urban subjects. Based on his research, Bates (1966) and Williams and Bates (1970) questioned why urban Blacks and not rural Blacks were so highly represented in the drug using group. O'Donnell et al. (1976) found the variable of residence in a large city until age 18 to be in direct proportion to greater use of drugs.

A different type of finding by Chein (1964) was that boys from neighborhoods where drugs were most prevalent held the most tolerant attitudes toward drugs and users but were least likely to possess correct information about drugs and their consequences. Among military drug abusers, Nail et al. (1974) concluded that many Blacks grow up in neighborhood subcultures full of street scenes and vernacular common to drug using groups. Illicit drug use in the military may not be a new experience but rather an extension of established subcultural patterns.

Several studies identified residential mobility as a commonality of stress for Black addicts. Abrams' (1967) study suggested that the liability to addiction seemed fairly high among male, non-white young persons. One source of this liability was social marginality felt by the addicts. These persons live in Chicago in areas that had a long history of Black settlement and had the most extensive internal migration. Ball et al. (1966) studied a large sample of incarcerated, addicted adults in Lexington. He found that Black addicts were from more migrant families than were whites. Intergenerational migration was twice as frequent among Blacks as contrasted to whites.

Within the Black community, religion, churches, and social

organizations have held an honored and valued position. Adolescent non-users of drugs reported themselves as allied with organized community programs and groups to a greater extent than did drug users. They were also found to more likely be engaged in sports activities and less likely to be engaged in purely social activities than did users. There is data to suggest that a youngster's early involvement in religious church activities may have some deterring effect on drug use (Globetti and Brigance, 1974; Craig and Brown, 1975).

## VALUES

Many American Blacks hold the middle-class values normative to the society. Based on a study of high school students, one investigation contended that middle-class Blacks made a more conscious effort to adhere to middle-class norms than did whites (Globetti and Brigance, 1974). Blacks rated higher than whites the terminal values of a comfortable life and equality. They were relatively less alienated from, and more concerned with, what are generally considered middle-class achievement oriented values than were white addicts (Miller et al., 1973). Based on interview data, a large majority of addicts noted specific material things and status considerably out of their reach. Their drive for vertical mobility was strong. The investigator concluded that the individual addict is overwhelmed with the necessity to "shut out" certain aspects of reality which are believed to be unattainable, therefore intolerable to him. Drug addiction is one of the defenses he uses to deal with the intolerable existance (Abrams et al., 1968).

Along with religion and middle-class values, many Black American families have believed that an education was the route to a better life and a step up the socioeconomic ladder. For many Blacks involved with drug use, their aspirations were thwarted.

## EDUCATION

Evidence supports the fact that for a large percentage of known adolescent drug abusers, unsuccessful school experiences have been the norm. Some of the more common problems have been: dropout; conflict with school personnel; skill deficiencies and difficulty in meeting school expectations.

Halikas (1976) reported that among Black, male drug users, more than 80% acknowledged at least some school problems prior to the age of 12 and 90% from the age 12 to 14; 90% acknowledged truancy beginning at about the seventh grade; about 80% had dropped out of formal schooling at some point during their childhood; about 33% had school change based on disciplinary problems; 81% had trouble with school authorities which led to 65% of the study population being suspended. Young persons generally begin their school career with high expectations, enthusiasm and positive attitudes toward the educational experience. In one study, older adolescent drug users reported better school adjustment; fewer difficulties with teachers and regarded school more favorably than did white users (Nail et al., 1974). In a different study group of Black adolescent drug users and non-users, 75% of both groups liked school and described themselves as good students. However, the drug users were significantly more likely to be school dropouts than were non-users (Craig and Brown, 1975). In New York City, non-addicts had been significantly more successful in school, 62% were high school graduates versus 32% of the addicts (Glasen et al., 1971).

A notable percentage of Black drug users were encouraged or exercised choice in terminating their formal schooling. Among adult drug users, they appear to have dropped out of school around 10th grade (Lander and Lander, 1967; Levi and Seborg, 1972). In a different study, Waldorf (1973) reported that an important factor in long abstention from drugs was neither class position nor ethnicity, but rather education. Persons who remained in high school had longer abstinences than those who dropped out.

In sum, a significant number of Black persons who have become drug abusers have had difficulties and interruptions in their efforts to receive formal schooling.

## CONCLUSIONS

Most of the cited variables place negative stress on Black families and ill equip the child in becoming fortified for handling developmental tasks of adolescence. Unstable home environments cannot provide the security and support a child needs to learn coping behaviors. Lack of employment degrades and erodes self-esteem. Families trapped in their struggle to meet basic survival needs, such as food, shelter and clothing may have little energy left to be a "good," responsive, nurturing parent. Being thwarted in an effort to attain middle-class values breeds frustration frequently ventilated in unproductive ways. Absence of a high school diploma limits access to employment and upward mobile opportunities. In the Black community, the church has not been fully exploited as a resource for families. Findings presented in this paper support the notion of family as having great influence on the lives and behavior of its young members. Norem-Hebeisen and Hedin (p. 28) issue the challenge for attempting to control some of the stressful conditions that occur in the early period of people's lives. "If we are to prevent alcohol and drug abuse and other problem behavior among youth, we need to maintain healthy balanced conditions and reduce exposure to harmful influences. We must attempt to decrease physical and emotional stress and increase a wide range of coping skills. We must also create and maintain healthy, constructive environments and social situations. By maximizing the survival, maintenance, and healthy growth of individuals and groups, we can reduce the likelihood of problem behavior."

## IMPLICATIONS FOR PREVENTION
## OF BLACK ADOLESCENT DRUG USE

The family nurtures and socializes its young members. A vast amount of public and private resources go into the control and treatment of drug abuse problems *after* they have been identified as such. It would be more cost effective to focus and channel resources in support of families. This would be primary prevention. It is more manageable to resolve marital conflict than to salvage the child who grows up to become a hard core drug addict.

A guiding principle for primary prevention with Black families is the value of starting where the person is. This means providing concrete services, social provisions and support as the young families define their needs.

Two underutilized resources that could provide help in strengthening young Black families are the school and the church. The drop out rate for consumers of both institutions suggests that services may not be meeting the needs of their constituencies. In keeping with these two institutions' missions, there are roles each can carry in helping families function in a manner that will prevent or reduce adolescent drug abuse.

In the broader social scheme, there is absence of a unified national family policy. Until the American family is politically viewed on the level of national defense and football, families and children will continue to suffer great disparity in the distribution of resources accessible to them. The family as the focus in primary prevention of adolescent drug abuse is a rational and efficient approach. In Blum's (1980) elegant argument on behalf of families, he stated "the most constant and intensive drug abuse prevention 'program' going is the daily life of the American family" (p. 110).

## REFERENCES

Abrams, A., Gagnon, J. H., and Levin, J. J. Psychosocial Aspects of Addiction. *American Journal of Public Health.* 1968, 58(11): 2142-2155.

Austin, G., Johnson, B., Carroll, E., and Lettieri, D. (eds.) *Research Issues 21, Drugs and Minorities.* National Institute on Drug Abuse, U.S. Department of Health, Education and Welfare, Public Health Service. 1977.

Ball, J. C. and Bates, W. M. Migration and Residential Mobility of Narcotic Drug Addicts. *Social Problems.* 1966, 14(1): 56-69.

Bates, W. M. Narcotics, Negroes and The South. *Social Forces.* 1966, 45(1): 61-67.

Bates, W. M. Occupational Characteristics of Negro Addicts. *International Journal of The Addictions.* 1968, 3(2): 345-350.

Blum, R. H. An Argument For Family Research. in Ellis, B. G. (ed.) *Drug Abuse From The Family Perspective: Coping Is a Family Affair.* Rockville, Maryland: U.S. Department of Human Services. National Institute on Drug Abuse. 1980, Chap. 10. pp. 104-116.

Brotman, R., and Freedman, A. *A Community Mental Health Approach to Drug Addiction.* Washington, D. C.: Government Printing Office, 1968.

Callan, J. P. and Patterson, C. D. Patterns of Drug Abuse Among Military Inductees. *American Journal of Psychiatry.* 1973, 130(3): 260-264.

Census Bureau, "Marital Status and Living Arrangements: March 1981." *New York Times* August 9, 1982, 9B.

Chambers, C. D. Some Epidemiological Considerations of Onset of Opiate Use in The United States, in Josephson, E. and Carroll, E. E. (eds.) *Drug Use: Epidemiological Approaches.* Washington, D.C.: Hemisphere Publishing, 1974, 66-81.

Chambers, C. D., Hinesley, R. K., and Moldestad, M. Narcotic Addiction in Females: A Race Comparison. *International Journal of The Addictions.* 1970, 5(2): 257-278.

Chein, I. Narcotics Among Juveniles in Cavan, R. (ed.) *Readings in Juvenile Delinquency.* New York: J. B. Lippincott. 1964, 237-252.

Craig, S. R. and Brown, Barry S. Comparison of Youthful Heroin Users and Non-users From One Urban Community. *International Journal of The Addictions.* 1975, 10(1): 53-64.

Force, E. E. and Millar, J. W. An Epidemiological and Ecological Study of Risk Factors for Narcotics Overdose: Retrospective Study of Psychosocial Factors. *International Journal of The Addictions* 1974, 9(3): 481-487.

Glaser, D., Lander, B., and Abbott, W. Opiate Addicted and Non-Addicted Siblings in a Slum Area. *Social Problems.* 1971, 18(4): 510-521.

Globetti, G., and Brigance, R. S. Rural Youth and The Use of Drugs, in Singh, J. M., Lal, H. eds. *New Aspects of Analytical and Clinical Toxicology.* New York: Stratton, 1974 (4): 255-262.

Glynn, T. J. From Family to Peer: Transitions of Influence Among Drug-Using Youth, in

Lettieri, D. J. and Ludford, J. P. (eds.) *Drug Abuse and The American Adolescent.* NIDA Research Monograph 38. Rockville, Maryland: U.S. Department of Health and Human Services, 1981, pp. 57-81.

Goldberg, P. and Meyers, E. J. The Influence of Public Attitudes and Understanding on Drug Education and Prevention in Drug Abuse Council. (ed.) *The Facts About "Drug Abuse."* New York: Free Press, 1980, Chap. 4. 126-152.

Goldsmith, B., Capel, W., Waddell, K., and Stewart, G. Demographic and Sociological Implications in New Orleans: Implications for Consideration of Treatment Modalities, in Singh, J., Miller, L., and Lal, H. (eds.) *Drug Addiction: Clinical and Socio-Legal Aspects.* Mount Kisco, New York: Future Publishing, 1972, 137-152.

Halikas, J. A., Darvish, H. S., and Rimmer, J. D. The Black Addict: 1. Methodology, Chronology of Addiction and Overview of The Population. *American Journal of Drug and Alcohol Abuse,* 1976.

Helmer, J., and Vietriosz, T. *Drug Use, The Labor Market and Class Conflicts,* Washington, D.C.: The Drug Abuse Council, 1974.

Kandel, D. Convergences in Prospective Longitudinal Surveys of Drug Use in Normal Populations, in Kandel, D. B. (ed.) *Longitudinal Research and Drug Use; Empirical Findings and Methodological Issues.* Washington, D. C.: Hemisphere-Wiley, 1978, 3-38.

Levi, M., and Seborg, M. The Study of I.Q. Scores on Verbal vs. Nonverbal Tests and vs. Academic Achievement Among Woman Addicts from Different Racial and Ethnic Groups. *International Journal of the Addictions.* 1972, 7(3): 581-584.

Lander, B., and Lander, N. A Cross-Cultural Study of Narcotic Addiction in New York, in Vocational Rehabilitation Administration. *Rehabilitating The Narcotic Addict.* Washington, D.C.: Government Printing Office, 1967, 359-369.

Lukoff, I., and Brook, J. A Sociocultural Exploration of Reported Heroin Use, in Winick, C., ed. *Sociological Aspects of Drug Dependence.* Cleveland, Ohio: CRC Press, 1974, 35-56.

Manatt, M. *Parents, Peers and Pot.* Rockville, Maryland: U.S. Department of Health and Human Services. National Institute on Drug Abuse, 1982.

Mare, R. D., and Winship, C. *Changes In The Relative Labor Force Status of Black and White Youths: A Review of The Literature.* University of Wisconsin-Madison, Institute For Research on Poverty, Special Report Series, 1980.

Miller, J., Sensenig, J., Stocker, R., and Campbell, R. Value Patterns of Drug Addicts as a Function of Race and Sex. *International Journal of The Addictions.* 1973, 8(4): 589-598.

Nail, R. L., Gunderson, E. K., and Arthur, R. J. Black-White Differences in Social Background and Military Drug Abuse Patterns. *American Journal of Psychiatry.* 1974, 13(10): 1097-1102.

National Commission on Marihuana and Drug Abuse. *Drug Use in America: Problem in Perspective,* Second Report, Washington, D. C.; U.S. Government Printing Office, 1973.

National Institute on Drug Abuse. *A Guide to Multicultural Drug Abuse Prevention: Strategies,* 3. Rockville, Maryland: U.S. Department of Health and Human Services, 1981,

Norem-Hebeisen, A., and Hedin, D. Influences on Adolescent Problem Behavior: Causes, Corrections and Contexts, in National Institute on Drug Abuse. *Adolescent Peer Pressure: Theory, Correlates, and Program Implications for Drug Abuse Prevention.* Rockville, Maryland: U.S. Department of Health and Human Services, 1981, Chap. II. 21-46.

O'Donnell, J. A., Voss, H., Clayton, R., Slatin, G., and Room, R. *Men and Drugs: A Nationwide Survey.* NIDA Research Monograph, Rockville, Maryland: National Institute in Drug Abuse. 1976 (5).

Robins, L. N., and Murphy, G. E. Drug Use in a Normal Population of Young Negro Men. *American Journal of Public Health.* 1967, 57(9): 1580-1596.

Roebuck, J. B. The Negro Drug Addict As An Offender Type. *Journal of Criminal Law, Criminology and Police Science.* 1962, 53(1): 36-43.

Stenmark, D., Wacwitz, J., Pelfrey, M., and Dougherty, F. Substance Use Among Juvenile

Offenders: Relationships to Parental Substance Use and Demographic Characteristics. *Addictive Diseases.* 1974, 1(1): 43-54.

Stephens, R., and Slatin, G. The Street Addict Role: Toward a Definition of a Type, *Drug Forum.* 1974, 3(4): 375-389.

Taylor, R. J., Jackson, J. S., and Quick, A. D. "The Frequency of Social Support Among Black Americans: Preliminary Findings From The National Survey of Black Americans" *Urban Research Review,* 1982, 8(2):1.

Vaillant, G. E. A Twelve-Year Follow-up of New York Narcotic Addicts: III Some Social and Psychiatric Characteristics. *Archives of General Psychiatry,* 1966, 15(6): 599-609.

Varenhorst, B. The Adolescent Society, in National Institute in Drug Abuse, *Adolescent Peer Pressure: Theory, Correlates and Program Implications for Drug Abuse Prevention.* U.S. Department of Health and Human Services, 1981, Chap. I. 1-20.

Waldorf, D. *Careers in Dope.* Englewood Cliffs, New Jersey, 1973.

Williams, J. E. and Bates, W. M. Some Characteristics of Female Narcotic Addicts. *International Journal of The Addictions,* 1970, 5(2): 245-256.

# Hispanic Adolescents and Substance Abuse: Issues for the 1980s

Denise Humm-Delgado
Melvin Delgado

**ABSTRACT.** The purpose of this article is to provide an understanding of the present state of knowledge about the problem of substance abuse among Hispanic youth and to identify issues with which researchers, clinicians, administrators, and policy makers will have to deal in the coming decade. To do so, it will focus on five major areas: (1) the limitations of drug-related statistics; (2) demographic characteristics of Hispanics in the United States; (3) a review of the literature on Hispanic adolescent substance abuse; (4) factors inhibiting a comprehensive analysis of the problem, its treatment, and appropriate policies; and (5) issues for the 1980s.

## INTRODUCTION

Adolescence is a developmental state that is often categorized as unsettling and filled with conflict and rebellion. The manner and success in which these upheavals are handled will determine to a great extent one's functioning as an adult; the adolescent who attempts to resolve stage-related issues with substance abuse is faced with additional burdens to resolve.

The impact of substance abuse on the lives of adolescents and their families is tremendous in terms of physical, emotional, and material tolls. The adolescent who is abusing drugs and other substances stands a higher probability of not finishing school, suffering from a variety of illnesses, and getting involved in crime than his or her counterpart who does not abuse drugs and other substances.

Denise Humm-Delgado is with the Office of the Court-Monitor for Special Education in Boston, MA. Melvin Delgado is in the School of Social Work at Boston University, Boston, MA 02215. Reprint requests should be addressed to Melvin Delgado.

*71*

However, if the adolescents who are abusing drugs happen to be Black or Hispanic, additional problems emerge when compared with their white counterparts, since the impact of poverty and racism compounds these.

The purpose of this article is to provide an understanding of the present state of knowledge about the problem of substance abuse among Hispanic youth and to identify issues which researchers, clinicians, administrators, and policy makers will have to deal with in the coming decade. To do so, it will focus on five major areas: (1) the limitations of drug-related statistics; (2) demographic characteristics of Hispanics in the United States; (3) a review of the literature on Hispanic adolescent substance abuse; (4) factors inhibiting a comprehensive analysis of the problem, its treatment and appropriate policies; and (5) issues for the 1980s.

## Limitations of Drug-Related Statistics

Before proceeding to examine the literature on substance abuse and Hispanic adolescents, it is important to highlight the context in which statistics are generally gathered on people of color, i.e., racial and ethnic minorities. There are three primary factors that serve to distort statistics related to this population: (1) reliance on arrest and treatment data; (2) type of drug frequently focused on by enforcement and treatment programs; and (3) undercounting by the U.S. Census (Liyama, Nishi, and Johnson, 1976, p.4).

Arrest and treatment statistics very often reflect on overrepresentation of Hispanics and other people of color (DeFleur, 1975; Helmer and Vietoriz, 1974). This is the result of their geographical location (poverty neighborhoods), visibility (color), limited economic resources to buy drugs through legal means, and the presence of racism and classism in the criminal justice system (from enforcement to incarceration).

Treatment data, which are often used for research, also reflect a high proportion of people of color. Treatment programs funded through public funds are frequently targeted towards poor people and, as a result of this type of funding, are subject to public scrutiny. Poor people have few or no alternatives to these programs, particularly if ordered to use them by the courts. In contrast, middle and upper-class people have more options available to them, and as a result, it is more difficult to detect and record their substance abuse.

In similar fashion to the above issues, type of drug used will also serve to inflate or deflate statistics:

> Another possible distortion in the assessment of the extent of dangerous drug abuse by minorities may be due to use of illegal opiates among non-white, non-Anglo, and lower-class populations. Whites and middle-class drug users may be more involved with drugs that are available through legal medical sources . . . As a consequence, when minorities use drugs, they may be more likely than whites to come into conflict with the law (Liyama, Nishi, and Johnson, 1976, p.7).

Thus, individuals who can afford to purchase their drugs through legal sources (doctors) or illegal means that minimize exposure (e.g., using other people to obtain the drugs) will not be recorded in arrest and treatment statistics.

Finally, the undercounting by the United States Census of the actual number of people of color in the country, legal and illegal, reduces the overall reported size of their total population. When combined with the above factors, this serves to increase the relative number of reported substance abusers within this population (Liyama, Nishi, and Johnson, 1976, p.7).

## DEMOGRAPHIC CHARACTERISTICS OF HISPANICS IN THE UNITED STATES

As already mentioned, statistics related to people of color must be closely examined prior to their use. This is not only applicable to substance abuse statistics but also to United States population statistics. Nevertheless, there are several sources of statistics regarding population size that do reflect to a great extent the actual numbers and characteristics of Hispanics in the United States. The importance of these demographic data cannot be underestimated, particularly as they relate to statistics on substance abuse among Hispanic adolescents.

Hispanics number approximately nineteen million with Mexican-Americans, Puerto Ricans, and Cubans representing the three largest groups (Peirce and Hagstrom, 1979, p. 549). These groups are increasing in size at a very rapid pace—during the 1970s the Hispanic population increased by thirty-three percent, three times the rate of Blacks and six times that of whites (McAdoo, 1982).

Estimates also show that Hispanics can be expected to surpass Blacks as the nation's largest minority within the next decade (*Time,* 1978).

Hispanics are a very young group, averaging twenty-three years of age—two years younger than Blacks and eight years younger than the national average (*N.Y. Times,* 1979). Hispanics consist primarily of young children and early adolescents with forty-three percent of the population under the age of nineteen, compared to forty percent for Blacks and thirty percent for the United States as a whole (U.S. Dept. of Commerce, 1981).

Hispanics are primarily urban-based (eighty-five percent compared to sixty-five percent for the nation) (Peirce and Hagstrom, 1979, p. 550), and are concentrated in the following areas:

> The Mexican Americans are largely concentrated in Texas, Arizona, and California and, to a lesser extent, are found in Colorado, New Mexico, and Illinois. The Puerto Rican-origin people are largely in New York City and adjacent areas of New Jersey; minor settlements are found in Illinois and California. The Cuban-descent population is concentrated in Florida, with minor settlements in the New York metropolitan area and California. Persons of Central and South American origin are found largely in New York and California. Substantial overlapping is found only in California and New York. Other states that contain many members of any one group tend to have only small pockets of other Spanish-American groups (Jaffe, Cullen, and Boswell, 1980, p.28).

In summary, Hispanics constitute a large and growing population in the United States, consisting of a high percentage of children, and generally residing in urban areas (Garcia, 1981).

### Review of the Literature

An extensive review of the literature published between 1970 and 1982 revealed that several authors have considered the issue of substance abuse among Hispanic adolescents. It is difficult to find major conclusive findings or theories that hold true throughout the literature, and it is clear that not only the etiology of substance abuse but also treatment methods for it need further study. In fact, many authors recommend that there be such further study.

The topics on which the literature focuses will be summarized below. The summary will delineate the groups, substances, settings, and geographical regions studied, as well as the findings about the characteristics and situations of the youth, and treatment issues that are presented.

*Groups Studied:* Hispanic groups studied in the literature vary, with some authors categorizing their study group as simply "Hispanic" (Jackson et al., 1981; Joseph, 1973; Kandel, Single, and Kessler, 1976; Rubio, 1980). One can of course often infer the primary Hispanic group studied because of the part of the country in which the research subjects live. However, since other Hispanics besides the primary group frequently live in the same area, it is not wise to assume, for example, that a sample from the Southwest is composed of all Mexican-Americans. (It should also be noted that the term "Hispanic" is sometimes used in the literature simply to differentiate the primary Hispanic group studied from Hispanics with a lesser representation in the particular study [Dembo et al., 1979a; Perez et at., 1980]).

Mexican-Americans and Puerto Ricans (both residing in Puerto Rico and in the United States) have received approximately equal attention in the literature, while Cuban-Americans have received very little (Note 1). This is a striking finding in that Mexican-Americans represent sixty percent of the Hispanic population, compared to ten percent for Puerto Ricans and five percent for Cuban-Americans (Peirce and Hagstrom, 1979, p. 549). Therefore, size of the population has not determined the amount of research undertaken in the last twelve years.

*Substances Studied:* The literature deals with substance abuse among Hispanic youth using a variety of definitions of "substances," influenced by factors such as the author's perception of the magnitude of the problem with a certain substance or substances for the sample studied, the substance use patterns of clientele in the particular treatment setting, or the wish to define abuse broadly (often for exploratory purposes). The choice of substances studied ranges from only narcotics (Amsel et al., 1971; Joseph, 1973; Zahn and Ball, 1972) through a variety of licit and illicit "drugs" (Crowther, 1972; Curtis and Simpson, 1976; Jimenez, 1980; Page, 1980). Many studies include or focus upon alcohol use (Dembo et al., 1979; Dembo et al., 1979a; DiBartolomeo, 1980; Nuttall and Nuttall, 1981; Padilla et al., 1979; Perez et al., 1980) while others include cigarettes as well as alcohol (Guinn, 1975; Jackson, 1981;

Kandel, Single, and Kessler, 1976; Robles, Martinez, and Moscoso, 1980). Inhalant abuse is also receiving attention, with a frequent
focus on Mexican-American adolescents (Dworkin and Stephens,
1980; Padilla et al., 1979; Perez et al., 1980; Rubio, 1980; Stybel,
Allen, and Lewis, 1976; Stybel, 1977).

Conclusive evidence does not exist regarding exactly which
substances the youth of each of the Hispanic groups uses, in what
patterns, or as compared to other ethnic-racial groups. For example, it is not known whether Hispanics have a greater tendency
than others to use heroin. However, the usage pattern with the most
corroboration in recent research literature seems to be the high use
of inhalants among Mexican-American adolescents as compared to
other adolescents (Padilla et al., 1979; Perez et al., 1980; Stybel,
Allen, and Lewis, 1976; Stybel, 1977). Besides research studies,
Dworkin and Stephens (1980) have also proposed a theoretical
model to help understand the problem and Rubio (1980) has discussed the possible contributions of community based organizations
to alleviating the problem.

*Research Settings:* Research settings are about evenly distributed
among samples in treatment, schools, and other community settings. Studies that deal with clients in treatment, either inpatient or
outpatient, include Amsel et al. (1971), Crowther (1972), Curtis
and Simpson (1976), Jimenez (1980), Joseph (1973), Page (1980),
Santisteban and Szapocznik (1982), and Zahn and Ball (1972).
Dembo et al. (1979 and 1979a) conducted research at the junior high
school level, while high schools were the settings used by Guinn
(1975), Kandel, Single, and Kessler (1976), Nuttall and Nuttall
(1981), Robles, Martinez, and Moscoso (1980), and Velez-Santori
(1981). Jackson et al. (1981) did research with youth of elementary
through high school ages, using samples obtained both from schools
and by outreach by community based organizations. Other community research settings include housing projects (Padilla et al.,
1979; Perez et al., 1980); a youth center (DiBartolomeo, 1980); and
a Youth Corps program in a school (Stybel, Allen, and Lewis,
1976; Stybel, 1977). By far the most frequently used data collection
method is surveys using interviews or self-administered question-
naires.

*Geographical Locations Studied:* Almost all regions of the United
States have received some attention in the research literature on substance abuse among Hispanic adolescents, even if the Hispanic
youth were only part of a broader sample, and one article utilizes

nationwide data (Curtis and Simpson, 1976). However, certain locations have been the setting for research more than others: New York, especially New York City (Amsel et al., 1971; Dembo et al., 1979 and 1979a; Joseph, 1973; Kandel, Single, and Kessler, 1976; Velez-Santori, 1981); Texas (Crowther, 1972; Guinn, 1975; Rubio, 1980; Stybel, Allen, and Lewis, 1976; Stybel, 1977); California, particularly East Los Angeles (Bloom and Padilla, 1979; Crowther, 1972; Padilla et al., 1979; Perez et al., 1980; Rubio, 1980). Puerto Rico has also been the site of a fair amount of research (Nuttall and Nuttall, 1981; Robles, Martinez, and Moscoso, 1980; Velez-Santori, 1981; Zahn and Ball, 1972).

*Characteristics and Situations:* Some findings in the literature regarding the characteristics and situations of Hispanic youth who abuse substances reflect a fair amount of attention and agreement. The lack of success or interest in school is seen as associated with various types of substance abuse (Dembo et al., 1979; Guinn, 1975; Nuttall and Nuttall, 1981; Perez et al., 1980; Santisteban and Szapocznik, 1982). Several authors agree that male adolescents generally tend to engage in substance use and abuse more than female adolescents (DiBartolomeo, 1980; Guinn, 1975; Nuttall and Nuttall, 1981; Page, 1980; Perez et al., 1980; Robles, Martinez, and Moscoso, 1980). Usage of certain drugs are seen generally to increase with age (Curtis and Simpson, 1976; Padilla et al., 1979; Perez et al., 1980). The peer groups is quite often cited as either reinforcing or dissuading substance use and abuse (DiBartolomeo, 1980; Guinn, 1975; Mata, 1978; Perez et al., 1980; Robles, Martinez, and Moscoso, 1980; Stybel, 1977). Additionally, receiving by far the most attention is the effect of the family relationship (Dembo et al., 1979; DiBartolomeo, 1980; Guinn, 1975; Jimenez, 1980; Nuttall and Nuttall, 1981; Page, 1980; Puyo, 1980; Robles, Martinez, and Moscoso, 1980; Santisteban and Szapocznik, 1982).

An issue that has received little attention in research and other literature is the effect of acculturation on substance use and abuse. A notable exception is an article about Cuban-Americans (Santisteban and Szapocznik, 1982) which uses information gained in an Hispanic family guidance center to propose hypotheses regarding acculturation and substance abuse. They describe the detrimental effect on the adolescent when a gap forms between the youth who acculturates and rejects parental authority and the parent who does not acculturate, resulting in neither parents nor children retaining a desirable "bicultural" approach to life.

*Treatment Issues:* The literature also gives very little in-depth attention to treatment methods or outcomes and there is no widely-accepted and successful treatment approach delineated. Rather, the literature focuses more upon identifying and describing samples who use or abuse substances. Yet several authors do at least suggest treatment principles or directions based upon their research, program experience, or theoretical work.

The need to develop programs based upon a knowledge of the particular population to be served is emphasized by Dembo et al. (1979), Guinn (1975), Jackson et al. (1981), Jimenez (1980), Page (1980), and Santisteban and Szapocznik (1982). Differential diagnosis leading to different treatment plans is suggested for the "social," "moderate," and "chronic" inhalant abuser (Stybel, Allen, and Lewis, 1976; Stybel, 1977). The importance of considering the role of the family in treatment or prevention is cited by Jimenez (1980), Padilla et al. (1979), and Santisteban and Szapocznik (1982).

Preventive or educational approaches that utilize the environment, such as increasing peer sanctions against substance use or abuse, are suggested by several authors in a variety of forms (DiBartolomeo, 1980; Dembo et al., 1979a; Rubio, 1980; Santisteban and Szapocznik, 1982; Stybel, Allen, and Lewis, 1976). In addition, when treatment or rehabilitation is necessary, alternatives to traditional therapy, which may be culturally unacceptable because of emphases such as group confrontation or the family's pathology, are provided by Jimenez (1980) and Santisteban and Szapocznik (1982), the latter authors describing a comprehensive model on which they are gathering outcome data.

## Factors Inhibiting a Comprehensive Analysis

The review of the literature on substance abuse among Hispanic adolescents highlights three important factors that make a comprehensive analysis of substance abuse among Hispanic adolescents difficult, if not impossible, at this time: (1) lack of certain research on this population; (2) lack of models that take into consideration cultural factors in examining or treating substance abuse; and (3) the frequent use of the term "Hispanic" to categorize all people of Spanish heritage, regardless of country of origin. A fourth important factor is that Hispanics are often subsumed in a "minority" category along with other racial and cultural groups. These factors make it difficult to develop prevention and treatment programs or social policies that effectively target and impact Hispanic adolescents who are substance abusers. The four factors are discussed below.

*Lack of Necessary Research:* As stated earlier, the review of the literature on Hispanic adolescents and substance abuse published within the last twelve years reveals several authors' interest in the topic. However, the literature unfortunately is not sufficiently extensive to allow many comparisons within and between Hispanic groups.

Analysis is further complicated due to a wide variation in the definitions of substance abuse and the different types and combinations of substances studied (Dworkin and Stephens, 1980; Guinn, 1975; Mata, 1978; Page, 1980; Perez et al., 1980; Puyo, 1980; Rubio, 1980). Studies also use not-comparable samples or methods and, even when several studies focus on one Hispanic group, different geographical settings or time frames restrict reliable comparisons. For example, the literature on Puerto Rican adolescents generally focuses on Puerto Ricans in either Puerto Rico or New York City, two geographical settings that represent very different environments.

It is also possible that the adolescent population in general may pose certain research constraints in that parental consent may be required but not forthcoming. Also, the reliance on treatment samples and school samples may produce findings not generalizable to the whole population, since the former may include primarily severely involved substance abusers or those identified by the courts, while the latter may exclude those who are already school drop-outs or absentees because of substance abuse.

*Cultural Model:* As noted by Santisteban and Szapocznik (1982), regardless of Hispanic origin, there are two basic tenets that cut across the Hispanic experience: (1) the importance of the family and (2) the challenges and problems associated with cultural adaptation. The authors conclude that these should play a prominent role in the conceptualization of prevention and treatment models focused on Hispanics.

Nevertheless, the literature notes few, if any, prevention and treatment programs that are based upon Hispanic cultural values (Szapocznik, Scopetta, and King, 1978). With the possible exception of Hispanic agencies (Rubio, 1980), most organizations dealing with drug abuse and addiction issues are not sensitized to the importance of culture in research, identification, assessment, and treatment of Hispanic adolescents. An excellent example of this is the tendency on the part of programs to neglect the importance of Hispanic natural support systems such as the extended family and religious organizations (Delgado and Humm-Delgado, 1982; Mannino and Shore, 1979). Intake forms and records are frequently limited to recording information pertaining to nuclear families and exclude extended family members or neighbors, and religion is also given little attention. However, religion can play a prominent part in the success or failure of services for Hispanic adolescents from various countries of origin. Consequently, programs that are not based upon cultural considerations experience failure to attract and keep Hispanic adolescents in treatment. Statistics on who is in treatment and on treatment outcomes, in turn, are biased.

Perez et al. (1980) note that the role of acculturation in increasing or decreasing substance abuse among Hispanic youth has not received in-depth or systematic investigation and that the complexity of studying acculturation cannot be minimized. The concept of acculturation covers a wide range of variables, with language abilities (Spanish/English) being just one type. Therefore, if one applies the concept of acculturation to substance abuse among Hispanic adolescents, it is necessary to operationalize it also to take into account culturally relevant behavior and values.

*The Label "Hispanic":* The limitations inherent in utilizing terms such as "Hispanic" and "Latino" in assessing community needs and making projections cannot be ignored. These terms have the advantage of grouping together people who share some degree of culture, language, and historical roots. However, for those who are knowledgeable of the differences that exist within and between Spanish-speaking groups, it quickly becomes apparent that classification into a major group tends to ignore major differences (Humm-Delgado and Delgado, forthcoming). Generally, these differences can be grouped into four categories: (1) different socioeconomic background and status; (2) degree and extent of influence of Spanish, African, and Indian backgrounds; (3) legal status in the United States (Crewdson, 1979, 1979a, 1979b, Ranklin, 1980); and (4) degree of acculturation to the United States. Consequently, ignoring how one defines the term "Hispanic" may very well result in comparing, for example, a Puerto Rican adolescent born and raised in the United States with a recently immigrated Costa Rican adolescent. Both may be classified as "Hispanic." Nevertheless, they may have more differences than commonalities (LeVine and Padilla, 1980).

In addition, the operational definition of "Hispanic" may be based upon any combination of a variety of criteria that may cast some doubt on the comparability of samples, since even *within* one subgroup of Hispanics, different criteria will tend to include or exclude certain individuals. Some of the most commonly used criteria include: country of origin, primary language, surname, country of origin of parents, location of birth, and self-disclosure (Vasquez and Uhlig, 1978). These criteria will influence the generalizability of findings (Hays-Bautista, 1980; Roberts and Lee, 1980).

*The Label "Minority":* The propensity to categorize Hispanics and other groups of people of color into a category of "minority" is fraught with limitations. Invariably, Blacks and Hispanics are grouped together when there is not a sufficiently large sample to warrant development of separate categories (Mandel, 1980; Lipscomb, 1971). Although the argument for combining these two groups is based upon similarity of socioeconomic status and other important variables such as geographical location, such actions take a simplistic approach to data collection and analysis; important cultural and linguistic differences are not considered by researchers who use this categorization.

## ISSUES FOR THE 1980s

The decade of the 1980s should prove to be of tremendous importance for Hispanics in the United States, in large part because it will be a period in which millions of Hispanic children enter adolescence and adulthood. In examining the major issues confronting Hispanic adolescents who are substance abusers, several can be identified, which can be grouped into five categories: (1) demographic projections; (2) research; (3) prevention; (4) treatment; and (5) policy.

*Demographic Projections:* The 1980s will witness the continued expansion of the Hispanic population in the United States; projections on the total size of this population range from twenty-five to thirty million for the 1980s, with the increase the result of increased birth rates and immigration (LeVine and Padilla, 1980; *New York Times,* 1982). It has been noted that the Hispanic birth rate is seventy-five percent greater than the national average (*New York Times,* 1982) and the number of Hispanic children can be expected to continue increasing at a rapid pace, with the adolescent population being similarly affected. The impact of substance abuse on the current and future population of adolescents must be seriously considered by researchers, clinicians, administrators, and policy makers.

*Research:* The role of research in the prevention and treatment of Hispanic adolescent substance abuse should increase in prominence in the 1980s. The knowledge gained through carefully conducted investigation will provide important answers concerning the etiology of the problem as well as its solutions and prevention. Research conducted in the 1980s should address the following research issues that became evident in the 1970s:

1. More studies are needed in non-treatment, non-court, and non-prison related settings to determine accurate substance prevalence. In addition, researchers should develop highly innovative techniques such as those developed by Bloom and Padilla (1979) in which they used adolescent peer interviewers.
2. There should be more longitudinal studies to obtain an in-depth understanding of changes of patterns of use over time; these would allow researchers to hypothesize about the impact of the environment on substance abuse, e.g., substance availability, "fads," and regional shifts due to population shifts, to suggest three possible important dimensions of the problem.
3. Researchers should clearly define the variables that enter into the definitions of "Hispanic" or "minority." Failure to delineate these terms will seriously limit the generalizability of research findings.
4. There should be increased research activity regarding various Hispanic subgroups, e.g., Mexican-Americans, who have received a disproportionately low amount of research, and on cultural themes such as the influence of acculturation on substance abuse.

*Prevention:* A preventive orientation to the problem of substance abuse has received little attention, but it is seriously needed and should utilize a variety of approaches. However, in light of the projected Hispanic demographic trends, it seems wise to consider doing the following in the 1980s:

1. Investigate and support ways to interest Hispanic youth in schools at a very early age, including the upgrading of the school systems themselves and their relevance to the Hispanic groups they serve.
2. Those substance abuse program staff with successful program models should disseminate information widely, by description of models and research on outcomes.
3. Encourage schools to take the lead in prevention, research, and model building, since they provide some of the broadest and earliest access to Hispanic children and their families, i.e., before treatment is even an issue.
4. Hispanic natural support systems should be utilized in preventive approaches, e.g., religious organizations or the extended family can be educated to the realities of substance abuse in order to support adolescents in withstanding peer pressure to abuse substances.

*Treatment:* The need to develop treatment techniques and programs based upon cultural values should continue in the 1980s. More successful programs should be developed that identify the adolescent who abuses substances at an early stage; for those at an advanced stage, it is imperative that treatment models be developed that stress not only psychological changes but the environmental context in which the adolescent finds himself or herself. For example, vocational and educational programs should be offered. In essence, every effort should be made to provide the adolescent with an opportunity to be a contributing member of the family and community.

Treatment programs and models also should not neglect Hispanic natural support systems. In fact, programs should be closely linked to these systems; this approach serves both to utilize cultural strengths and reintegrate the adolescent who abuses substances into the Hispanic community.

*Policy:* Social policies directed at substance abuse should take into account substance abuse among Hispanic adolescents and stress the following issues:

1. There is a need for the examination and remediation of the environmental supports for illicit drug abuse so that not only the users' personal characteristics are the focus of policy. For example, how and why are some communities targeted for the

sale of illicit drugs and how does the easy availability of illicit drugs to Hispanic youth influence their drug use patterns?

2. Policy makers need to take into account demographic trends (number of children, urban-rural base, growing population, and areas of concentration) and reflect these trends in substance abuse policies for the 1980s. For example, program or research funding to areas with high numbers of Hispanics should include a requirement that some resources be used for this group.

3. Policies need to address subgroup differences, not just language, and require that funded programs do likewise.

4. The United States Census Bureau needs to develop ways to count Hispanics accurately. Without a sound understanding of their numbers and characteristics, it is virtually impossible to develop appropriate policies and programs.

5. Every effort should be made to employ Hispanics in key positions to assist Hispanic youngsters through culturally relevant service delivery and appropriate role modeling. A lack of Hispanic representation in key institutions such as schools does not provide Hispanics with important access to individuals with similar backgrounds and culture. Funding should be directed at this human resource development.

## CONCLUSION

The problem of substance abuse among Hispanic adolescents has been examined in terms of the present state of knowledge about the topic and issues that are yet to be understood and resolved in the 1980s. It was suggested that, although there is a good deal of interest in the problem as witnessed by the literature over the past twelve years, certain areas need further research. It was also suggested that attention to culture-specific programs and policies is needed, and recommendations for such programs and policies, as well as research, were made.

## REFERENCE NOTE

1. Our literature review found the following literature that deals with Puerto Ricans: Amsel et al., 1971; Curtis and Simpson, 1976; Dembo et al., 1979; Dembo et al., 1979a; DiBartolomeo, 1980; Jimenez, 1980; Nuttall and Nuttall, 1981; Puyo, 1980; Robles, Martinez, and Moscoso, 1980; Velez-Santori, 1981; Zahn and Ball, 1972. Several authors fo-

cused on Mexican-Americans: Bloom and Padilla, 1979; Crowther, 1972; Curtis and Simpson, 1976; Dworkin and Stephens, 1980; Guinn, 1975; Mata, 1978; Padilla et al., 1979; Perez et al., 1980; Stybel, Allen, and Lewis, 1976; Stybel, 1977). Literature focusing on Cuban-Americans included: Page, 1980; Santisteban and Szapocznik, 1982.

# REFERENCES

*Age, Sex, Race, and Spanish Origin of the Population by Regions, Divisions, and States: 1980.* U.S. Dept. of Commerce, Bureau of the Census, May 1981.

Amsel, Z. et al. The use of the narcotics register for follow-up of a cohort of adolescent addicts. *International Journal of the Addictions,* 1971, 6, 225-239.

Bloom, D. and Padilla, A. M. A peer interviewer model in conducting surveys among Mexican-American youth. *Journal of Community Psychology,* 1979, 7, 129-136.

Birth Rate Highest for Latins in U.S. *New York Times,* May 26, 1982, C4.

Crewdson, J. M. Thousands of aliens held in virtual slavery in U.S. *New York Times,* October 19, 1980, 1, 58.

Crewdson, J. M. Female illegal aliens often virtual slaves. *New York Times,* October 23, 1980, A18. (a)

Crewdson, J. M. Illegal aliens are bypassing farms for higher pay of jobs in the cities. *New York Times,* November 10, 1980, A1, D9. (b)

Crowther, B. Patterns of drug use among Mexican Americans. *International Journal of the Addictions,* 1972, 7, 637-647.

Curtis, B. and Simpson, D. D. Demographic characteristics of groups classified by patterns of multiple drug abuse: A 1969-1971 sample. *International Journal of the Addictions,* 1976, 11, 161-173.

DeFleur, L. B. Biasing influences on drug arrest records: Implications for deviance research. *American Sociological Review,* 1975, 40, 88-103.

Delgado, M., and Humm-Delgado, D. Natural support systems: Source of strength in Hispanic communities. *Social Work,* 1982, 27, 83-89.

DiBartolomeo, J. J. *A descriptive study of the problem drinking behavior among Spanish-speaking youth of Puerto Rican heritage.* Doctoral Dissertation. University of Maryland, 1980.

Dembo, R. et al. Self-concept and drug involvement among urban junior high school youths. *International Journal of the Addictions,* 1979, 14, 1125-1144.

Dembo, R. et al. Ethnicity and drug use among urban junior high school youths. *International Journal of the Addictions,* 1979, 14, 557-568. (a)

Dworkin, A. G., and Stephens, R. C. Mexican-American adolescent inhalant abuse: A proposed model. *Youth and Society,* 1980, 11, 493-506.

Fitzpatrick, J. *Puerto Rican Americans: The meaning of migration to the mainland.* Englewood Cliffs, N.J.: Prentice-Hall, Inc., 1971.

Garcia, J. A. Hispanic migration: Where they are moving and why. *Agenda,* 1981, 11, 14-17.

Guinn, R. Characteristics of drug use among Mexican-American students. *Journal of Drug Education,* 1975, 5, 235-241.

Hayes-Bautista, D. E. Identifying Hispanic populations: The influence of research methodology upon public policy. *American Journal of Public Health,* 1980, 70, 353-356.

Helmer, J., and Vietorisz, T. *Drug use, the market and class conflict.* Washington, D.C.: The Drug Abuse Council, 1974.

Hispanic Americans soon the biggest minority. *Time,* October 16, 1978, 48-61.

Humm-Delgado, D., and Delgado, M. Assessing Hispanic mental health needs: Issues and recommendations. *Journal of Community Psychology,* forthcoming publication.

LeVine, E. S., and Padilla, A. M. *Crossing cultures in therapy: Pluralistic counseling for the Hispanic.* Monterey: Brooks/Cole, 1980.

Lipscomb, W. R. Drug use in a black ghetto. *American Journal of Psychiatry,* 1971, 127, 1166-1169.

Jackson, N. Age of initial drug experimentation among white and non-white ethnics. *International Journal of the Addictions,* 1981, 16, 1373-1386.

Jaffe, A. J., Cullen, R., and Boswell, T. D. *The changing demography of Spanish Americans.* New York: Academic Press, 1980.

Jimenez, D. R. A comparative analysis of the support systems of white and Puerto Rican clients in drug treatment programs. Saratoga, CA: Century Twenty-One Publishing, 1980.

Joseph, H. A probation department treats heroin addicts. *Federal Probation,* 1973, 37, 35-39.

Kandel, D., Single, E., and Kessler, R. C. The epidemiology of drug use among New York state high school students: Distribution, trends and change in rates of use. *American Journal of Public Health,* 1976, 66, 43-53.

Liyama, P., Nishi, S. M., and Johnson, B. D. *Drug use and abuse among U.S. minorities: An annotated bibliography.* New York: Praeger Publishers, 1976.

Mandel, J. Statistics blur miniority distinctiveness. *International Journal of the Addictions,* 1980, 15, 1297-1300.

Mannino, F. V. and Shore, M. F. Perceptions of social supports by Spanish-speaking youth with implications for program development. *Journal of School Health,* 1976, XLVI, 471-474.

Mata, A. G. *The drug street scene: An ethnographic study of Mexican youth in south Chicago.* Doctoral Dissertation, University of Notre Dame, 1978.

McAdoo, H. P. Demographic trends for people of color. *Social Work,* 1982, 27, 15-23.

*New York Times,* Hispanics fastest growing minority in U.S., February 18, 1979.

Nuttall, R. L., and Nuttall, E. V. A longitudinal study predicting heroin and alcohol use among Puerto Ricans. In A. J. Schecter, Ed. *Drug Dependence and Alcoholism, Vol. 2, Social & Behavorial Issues.* New York: Plenum Press, 1981.

Oscar, A. J. *Puerto Ricans and health: Findings from New York city.* New York: Fordham University Spanish Mental Health Research Center, 1978.

Padilla, E. R. et al. Inhalant, marijuana, and alcohol abuse among barrio children and adolescents. *International Journal of the Addictions,* 1979, 14, 945-964.

Page, J. B. The children of exile: Relationships between the acculturation process and drug use among Cuban youth. *Youth and Society,* 1980, 11, 431-447.

Peirce, N. R., and Hagstrom, J. The Hispanic community—a growing force to be reckoned with. *National Journal,* April 7, 1979, 548-555.

Perez, R. et al. Correlates and changes over time in drug and alcohol use within a barrio population. *American Journal of Community Psychology,* 1980, 8, 621-636.

Preble, E. Social and cultural factors related to narcotic use among Puerto Ricans in New York city. *International Journal of the Addictions,* 1966, 2, 30-41.

Puyo, A. M. *Family headship and drug addiction among male Puerto Rican youths: An investigation of quality of family life.* Doctoral Dissertation, Fordham University, 1980.

Rankin, D. Help available for aliens. *New York Times Week in Review Section,* October 18, 1980, 32.

Roberts, R. E., and Lee, E. S. Methodological issues in health care surveys of the Spanish heritage population. *American Journal of Public Health,* 1980, 70, 367-374.

Robles, R. A., Martinez, R. E., and Moscoso, M. R. Predictors of adolescent drug behavior: The case of Puerto Rico. *Youth and Society,* 1980, 6, 415-430.

Rubio, G. CBOs helping inhalant abusers. *Agenda,* 1980, 10, 9-11.

Santisteban, D., and Szapocznik, J. Substance abuse disorders among Hispanics: A focus on prevention. In R. M. Becerra, M. Karno, and J. I. Escobar, Eds. *Mental Health and Hispanic Americans Clinical Perspectives.* New York: Grune & Stratton, 1982, 83-100.

Stybel, L. J. Psychotherapeutic options in the treatment of child and adolescent hydrocarbon inhalers. *American Journal of Psychotherapy,* 1977, 31, 525-532.

Stybel, L. J., Allen, P., and Lewis, F. Deliberate hydrocarbon inhalation among low socioeconomic adolescents not necessarily apprehended by the police. *International Journal of the Addictions,* 1976, 11, 345-361.

Szapocznik, J., Scopetta, M. A., and King, O. E. Theory and practice in matching treatment to the special characteristics and problems of Cuban immigrants. *Journal of Community Psychology,* 1978, 6, 112-122.

Valle, M. *What holds Sami back?: A Study of Service Delivery in a Puerto Rican Community.* New York: Valle Associates, 1973.

Vasquez, A. G., and Uhlig, G. E. The Spanish-speaking of Chicago: Social service issues. *Social Perspectives,* 1978, 6, 25-29.

Velez-Santori, C. N. *Drug use among Puerto Rican youth: An exploration of generational status differences.* Doctoral Dissertation, Columbia University, 1981.

Zahn, M. A., and Ball, J. C. Factors related to cure of opiate addiction among Puerto Rican addicts. *International Journal of the Addictions,* 1972, 7, 237-245.

# Psychotropic and General Drug Use by Mentally Retarded Persons: A Test of the Status Model of Drug Use

Ann E. MacEachron

**ABSTRACT.** The proposed status model of drug use made differential predictions for use of general medications and psychotropic drugs on the basis of employment status, physical health status, mental status, and institutional status. The model was supported for a population of approximately 42,000 mentally retarded persons of all ages receiving services in one state and for a subgroup of approximately 7,000 adolescents. Theoretical and applied implications were discussed.

Drug use among adolescents is commonly thought of as the voluntary consumption of illicit drugs that change behaviors or moods. Heroin users are pictured as urban black males (e.g., Weppner, Wells, McBride, and Ladner, 1976), while users of marijuana, psychedelic drugs and, more recently, illicit prescription drugs are pictured as middle-class and upper-class suburban youth (e.g., Dembo, Schmeidler, and Koral, 1976). But the other side of the coin shows that some adolescent drug users, often judged to be mentally ill or mentally retarded, are given legal prescription drugs to change their behaviors or moods. Both groups use drugs to change

Ann E. MacEachron is associated with the Program Research Unit of the New York State Office of Mental Retardation and Developmental Disabilities, 44 Holland Avenue, Albany, NY 12229. She is also affiliated with Brandeis University and the Eunice Kennedy Shriver Center. Reprint requests should be addressed to the author.

their behaviors and moods and both groups are believed to have problems, but for very different reasons—one group because they use drugs, and the other group because they have mental problems. A solution for the former group is to take away drugs that change behaviors or moods, while a solution for the latter group is to give drugs that change behaviors or moods. The immediate focus of this paper is to describe drug use among the latter group, that is, adolescents who are mentally retarded and who take prescribed psychotropic drugs. The larger focus, however, is to reconceptualize the idea of drug use within a broader context of general drug use.

Psychotropic drugs are defined here "as prescription medications given for the purpose of producing beneficial changes in mood, thought processes, or behavior. They are classified as major tranquilizers, minor tranquilizers, anti-depressants, stimulants and sedative-hypnotics" (Lipman, DiMascio, Reatig and Kirson, 1978: 1437). Such drugs have been developed and used for treatment of mental illness only during the last twenty-five years. However, as Berger (1978:974) has pointed out: "The use of drug treatments for mental illness is not all positive: problems have arisen for patients, physicians, and society. The drugs are not ideal. Not all patients are helped, and many are only partially improved. Like other useful medications, the pharmacological agents used in mental illness can cause severe adverse reactions; some of the side effects are irreversible. Certain classes of drugs for psychiatric patients are toxic when taken in an overdose."

The original intent of psychotropic drugs was for the treatment of severe mental illness: schizophrenia, depression, and mania. Yet the promise of psychotropic drugs has seemed so great that they are used in a variety of situations for a number of problems beyond severe mental illness (Sprague and Baxley, 1978). For example, institutionalized mentally retarded persons with behavior problems— and not necessarily just those who are also mentally ill—are reported to be frequent users of psychotropic drugs. Studies of institutions for mentally retarded persons in the United States have found that between 45% and 60% of the residents receive psychotropic drugs (Lipman, 1970; DiMascio, 1975; Marker, 1975). Similar percentages have been reported for England (Kirman, 1976), New Zealand (Sewell and Werry, 1976) and Canada (Tu, 1979). Several of these studies also reported that residents were receiving more than the recommended doses and had been using such drugs continuously for a number of years; both factors increase substantially the chances of deleterious side effects (Sprague and Baxley, 1978; Berger, 1978). The relationship between psychotropic drug use and institutionalization has also been observed for a different population, the aged. Zawadski, Glazer, and Lurie (1978) found substantial differences in psychotropic drug use based on residential setting: 5 percent of drug expenditures for the non-institutionalized aged were for psychotropic drugs, 40 percent for the institutionalized aged, and 16 percent for the noninstitutional aged who were medically similar to the institutionalized aged. Zawadski et al. then suggested a "layering" model to describe prescription drug use: a baseline level of drug usage for the general population typically includes antacids, antiobiotics, analgesics, and vitamins; another "layer" is superimposed for people with chronic physical illnesses who tend to use such drugs as antihypertensives, diuretics, and antidiabetes medications; and among the institutionalized, another "layer" of psychotropic drugs is added.

The layering model of prescription drug use is useful in two respects: (1) it describes conceptually distinct types of drug use—normal baseline usage, general medication usage for physical health reasons, and psychotropic drug usage for mental reasons, and (2) it describes psychotropic drug use in context of the situation around the person and not just in terms of individual characteristics. There are three problems with this model, however: (1) it focuses only on the aged and is thus limited in generality, (2) it lacks an explanation of the dynamics that shift a person from a baseline level of drug use to additional superimposed layers of drug use, and (3) it links the conceptually separate issues of institutionalization and psychotropic drug use. Given the strengths and limitations of the layering model, another model of drug use may be developed. This proposed model is called a "status" model of prescription drug use.

The "status" model maintains the three distinct types of drug use of the layer model, but here they are thought of as three separate uses of drugs rather than superimposed layers. Thus, the drug use types may apply to the general population and not only to the aged. The status model also incorporates four dimensions of status to explain the dynamics underlying type of drug use: (1) employment status, (2) physical health status, and (3) mental status, and (4) institutional status. Employment status is perhaps the most important dynamic to incorporate because people who are employed are not prone to drug use beyond the baseline. Unemployment either causes or reflects an increased likelihood of physical health problems (Luft, 1978) and mental problems (Brenner, 1973; Berg and Hughes, 1979). As the presence of physical health problems leads to the use of general medications to ameliorate or control physical conditions, so it is expected that the presence of mental problems—be they psychiatric, psychological, or developmental—leads to the use of psychotropic drugs to ameliorate or control mental conditions. Thus, institutionalization per se, is not needed to explain type of drug use. Yet institutionalization is a supplemental concept to the other three statuses. If unemployed, there is a greater likelihood of drug use beyond the baseline for reasons of physical or mental problems; if the physical or mental problems are severe, then there is the likelihood of even greater drug use and a substantial likelihood of institutionalization. Institutionalization is generally considered to be the option of last choice and represents the inability or unwillingness of a single set of persons—be they parents, spouses, foster parents, or group home staff—to continue the support of the unemployed person in the community. This unemployed person is likely to be institutionalized when his or her physical problems result in functional dependence in daily living skills or when his or her mental problems result in behavior control problems. While institutionalization may well further aggravate these problems and increase drug usage, increasingly stringent admissions policies for institutions and increasingly available community services suggest that what admissions do occur will reflect rather severe problems for the unemployed person.

In sum, then, the status model is parsimonious in the number of concepts needed to explain the predictive dynamics underlying drug use. Unemployment encompasses most people who are prone to drug use—the urban black male, the middle and upper class adolescent, the aged, the physically and mentally disabled and the housewife. Physical and mental statuses then determine type of drug use, while severe physical and mental statuses determine substantial drug use and institutionalization in turn magnifies drug use.

The present study is a beginning attempt to test the proposed status model of drug use. It is hypothesized that:

1. Use of general medications will be associated with unemployment, physical disabilities, and dependent functioning in daily living skills.

2. Use of psychotropic drugs will be associated with unemployment, mental disabilities, and behavior control problems.
3. Use of general medications and psychotropic drugs will be associated with institutionalization.
4. Institutionalization will be more strongly associated with unemployment, dependent functioning in daily living skills, and behavior control problems than with such alternative explanations as age, gender, and ethnicity.
5. These hypotheses will predict equally well for the general population and the adolescent population.

As such, then, the status model is a generalizable model of drug use. While the present study only tests its utility among a population of mentally retarded persons receiving services in one state, it does provide at least one population perspective that if successful will suggest its potential utility for other population groups.

## METHODOLOGY

*Subjects.* The subjects were 41,643 mentally retarded persons between the ages of 1 and 94 who were receiving services in one large northeastern state from 1979 to 1981. The subgroup of adolescents consisted of 7,392 mentally retarded persons from age 13 to 21.

*Measures.* All subject information came from the state's management information system (Janicki and Jacobson, Note 1).

*Psychotropic drugs* included such drugs as mellaril, thorazine, stelazine, serentil, tofranil, sedatives, and stimulants. *General medications* included diabetic drugs, anti-convulsant drugs, cardiac drugs, and other prescribed medications. *Physical disabilities* included thirteen physical problems such as sensory, respiratory, cardiovascular, digestive, musculo-skeletal, hemic/lymphatic and neoplastic disease. *Multiple developmental disabilities* included mental retardation and the additional presence of autism, cerebral palsy, epilepsy, or neurological impairment. *Psychiatric disabilities* included nine problems such as organic brain syndrome, psychosis, neurosis, personality disorders, and psychophysiologic disorders. *Behavior control problems* included nineteen problems that would prohibit placement of the person in a less restrictive setting or constitute a partial barrier to the provision of services such as physical assaults on others, property destruction, firesetting, coercive sexual behavior, self-injurious action, hyperactivity, and stereotypic/repetitive movements. Currently *working* included six forms of work: sheltered workshop, work adjustment, sheltered employment, work experience program, competitive employment, and vocational education. *Institutional living* included all forms of congregate care in contrast to community living either independently, with family, in foster care, or in group homes. *Gender* was measured by a score of 0 indicating males and a score of 1 indicating females. *Ethnicity* was measured by a score of 0 indicating minorities and a score of 1 indicating whites. The above variables were measured as dichotomous variables where a score of 0 indicated the absence of the characteristic and a score of 1 indicated the presence of the characteristic: psychotropic drug use, general medication drug use, physical disabilities, multiple developmental disabilities, psychiatric disabilities, behavior control problems, being female, being of white ethnicity, currently working, and living in an institution.

*Independent functioning in daily living skills* was evaluated by a three-point scale (1 = dependent, 2 = needs training or supervision, 3 = independent) measuring toileting skills, eating skills, and dressing skills.

*Age* was measured in years.

The means and standards for each variable fo the population are shown in Table 1 and for adolescents alone in Table 2.

*Analysis.* The hypotheses were tested by the strength and direction of Pearson correlation coefficients and by multiple regression techniques. Age, gender, and ethnicity were included in the analysis as alternative explanations for institutionalization as well as for psychotropic and general medication use. The level of significance used throughout the study was p < .001.

## RESULTS

The utilization of general medications was 38% for the population and 33% for adolescents. The utilization of psychotropic drugs was 22% for the population and 16% for adolescents. Use of one type of drug did not appear to predicate the use of the other type of drug.

As expected for Hypothesis 1, use of general medications for the population (Table 1) and for adolescents (Table 2) was significantly associated with unemployment ($r_p = -.11$, $r_a = -.09$), the presence of physical disabilities ($r_p = .32$, $r_a = .32$), and multiple

TABLE 1

SIGNIFICANT (p < .001) PEARSON CORRELATIONS FOR THE POPULATION OF

MENTALLY RETARDED PERSONS IN ONE STATE (N=37,829 to 41,643)

| VARIABLES | (1) | (2) | (3) | (4) | (5) | (6) | (7) | (8) | (9) | (10) | (11) | (12) | (13) | (14) |
|---|---|---|---|---|---|---|---|---|---|---|---|---|---|---|
| 1. Psychotropic drugs | 1.00 | | | | | | | | | | | | | |
| 2. General medications | .07 | 1.00 | | | | | | | | | | | | |
| 3. Currently working | -.08 | -.11 | 1.00 | | | | | | | | | | | |
| 4. Institution living | .26 | .24 | -.35 | 1.00 | | | | | | | | | | |
| 5. Psychiatric disabilities | .22 | | .02 | .03 | 1.00 | | | | | | | | | |
| 6. Behavior control problems | .30 | .09 | -.15 | .29 | .15 | 1.00 | | | | | | | | |
| 7. Physical disabilities | | .32 | -.18 | .26 | | .07 | 1.00 | | | | | | | |
| 8. Multiple DD | | .36 | -.19 | .19 | .03 | .06 | .38 | 1.00 | | | | | | |
| 9. Toileting skills | .02 | -.21 | .39 | -.33 | .08 | -.05 | -.31 | -.35 | 1.00 | | | | | |
| 10. Eating skills | -.02 | -.21 | .39 | -.36 | .06 | -.07 | -.30 | -.33 | .82 | 1.00 | | | | |
| 11. Dressing skills | -.03 | -.21 | .44 | -.37 | .06 | -.10 | -.31 | -.35 | .79 | .77 | 1.00 | | | |
| 12. Age | .10 | .14 | .17 | .19 | | -.06 | .07 | -.14 | .22 | .20 | .19 | 1.00 | | |
| 12. Gender | | .06 | | .02 | -.03 | | .04 | | -.02 | | | .07 | 1.00 | |
| 14. Ethnicity | | .05 | .06 | .02 | -.04 | | .02 | -.04 | -.03 | .03 | .03 | .19 | .02 | 1.00 |
| MEAN | .22 | .38 | .25 | .44 | .11 | .47 | .50 | .34 | 2.50 | 2.50 | 2.30 | 32 | .45 | .82 |
| STANDARD DEVIATION | .41 | .48 | .44 | .50 | .31 | .50 | .50 | .47 | .74 | .68 | .70 | 17 | .50 | .38 |

## TABLE 2

SIGNIFICANT (p < .001) PEARSON CORRELATIONS FOR MENTALLY RETARDED

ADOLESCENTS (N=6,595 to 7,392)

| VARIABLES | (1) | (2) | (3) | (4) | (5) | (6) | (7) | (8) | (9) | (10) | (11) | (12) | (13) | (14) |
|---|---|---|---|---|---|---|---|---|---|---|---|---|---|---|
| 1. Psychotropic drugs | 1.00 | | | | | | | | | | | | | |
| 2. General medications | | 1.00 | | | | | | | | | | | | |
| 3. Currently working | -.04 | -.09 | 1.00 | | | | | | | | | | | |
| 4. Institution living | .20 | .24 | -.16 | 1.00 | | | | | | | | | | |
| 5. Psychiatric disabilities | .25 | -.08 | .05 | .04 | 1.00 | | | | | | | | | |
| 6. Behavior control problems | .32 | .06 | -.07 | .21 | .22 | 1.00 | | | | | | | | |
| 7. Physical disabilities | -.04 | .32 | -.12 | .29 | -.05 | .04 | 1.00 | | | | | | | |
| 8. Multiple DD | .05 | .43 | -.13 | .23 | | .05 | .43 | 1.00 | | | | | | |
| 9. Toileting skills | | -.33 | .20 | -.40 | .12 | | -.41 | -.41 | 1.00 | | | | | |
| 10. Eating skills | | -.32 | .19 | -.39 | .11 | | -.39 | -.40 | .83 | 1.00 | | | | |
| 11. Dressing skills | | -.32 | .23 | -.40 | .09 | -.02 | -.39 | -.41 | .81 | .79 | 1.00 | | | |
| 12. Age | .07 | | .23 | .07 | | | -.05 | -.07 | .14 | .13 | .14 | 1.00 | | |
| 13. Gender | -.06 | .04 | | | -.05 | | .07 | | -.05 | -.06 | -.07 | | 1.00 | |
| 14. Ethnicity | -.08 | | -.04 | | -.09 | -.08 | | -.03 | .05 | -.06 | .03 | | | 1.00 |
| MEAN | .18 | .33 | .06 | .42 | .12 | .47 | .50 | .43 | 2.30 | 2.40 | 2.10 | 18 | .41 | .73 |
| STANDARD DEVIATION | .36 | .47 | .23 | .49 | .32 | .50 | .50 | .49 | .79 | .72 | .73 | 3 | .49 | .44 |

developmental disabilities ($r_p$ = .36, $r_a$ = .43), and dependence in toileting skills ($r_p$ = −.21, $r_a$ = −.33), dependence in eating skills ($r_p$ = −.21, $r_a$ = −.32), and dependence in dressing skills ($r_p$ = −.21, $r_a$ = −.32). These six predictors accounted for a significant amount of variation in the use of general medications for the population (R = .42, $R^2$ = .17) and for adolescents (R = .47, $R^2$ = .22).

As expected for Hypothesis 2, use of psychotropic drugs for the population (Table 1) and for adolescents (Table 2) was significantly associated with unemployment ($r_p$ = −.08, $r_a$ = −.04), the presence of psychiatric disabilities ($r_p$ = .22, $r_a$ = .25), and the presence of behavior control problems ($r_p$ = .30, $r_a$ = .32). These three predictors accounted for a significant amount of variation in the use of psychotropic drugs for the population (R = .37, $R^2$ = .13), and for adolescents (R = .37, $R^2$ = .14).

As expected for Hypothesis 3, institutionalization in the population and for adolescents was associated with the use of general medications ($r_p$ = .24, $r_a$ = .24), and the use of psychotropic drugs ($r_p$ = .26, $r_a$ = .20).

As expected for Hypothesis 4, the likelihood of institutionalization within the population (Table 1) and for adolescents (Table 2) was not strongly associated with unemployment ($r_p$ = −.35, $r_a$ = −.16), dependent functioning in toileting skills ($r_p$ = −.33, $r_a$ = −.40), dependent functioning in eating skills ($r_p$ = −.36, $r_a$ = −.39), dependent functioning in dressing skills ($r_p$ = −.37, $r_a$ = −.40), and the presence of behavior control problems ($r_p$ = .29, $r_a$ = .21). These five predictors accounted for a significant amount of variation in the likelihood of institutionalization for the population (R = .52, $R^2$ = .27) and for adolescents (R = .51, $R^2$ = .26). In contrast, age, gender and ethnicity were less strongly associated with institutionalization and accounted for a lesser but still significant amount of variation for the population (R = .18, $R^2$ = .03) and for adolescents (R = .07, $R^2$ = .01). Relatedly, these three predictors accounted for a lesser amount of variation in the use of general medications for the population (R = .15, $R^2$ = .02, p < .001) and adolescents (R = .04, $R^2$ = .002 p > .01), and in the use of psychotropic drugs for the population (R = .10, $R^2$ = .01, p < .001) and adolescents (R = .15, $R^2$ = .02).

As expected for Hypothesis 5, the hypotheses derived from the status model of drug use were supported equally well for both the population and adolescents. That is, Hypotheses 1, 2, 3, and 4 were supported empirically for both groups.

## DISCUSSION

The status model of drug use was supported in predicting drug use and in distinguishing psychotropic drug use from use of general medications. While unemployment was related to greater use of both types of drugs, the presence of physical disabilities and dependent functioning in daily skills were strong predictors of the use of general medications and the presence of psychiatric disabilities and behavior control problems were strong predictors of the use of psychotropic drugs. Institutionalization was associated with greater use of both types of drugs, and especially well related to dependent functioning in daily living skills and behavior control problems. These findings occurred for both the general population of mentally retarded persons and for the group of adolescents.

From a conceptual perspective, the status model presents a parimonious model to explain drug use. The four status factors contained in the model—employment status, physical health status, mental status, and institutional status—both describe and predict drug use. While other situational and individual characteristics might well improve the predictive utility of the model, at least it has been demonstrated that this model is plausible. Moreover, as presented, the status model is presumed generalizable to and best tested in broadly defined populations. The current study only examined a population characterized by the developmental disability of mental retardation, a population particularly vulnerable to unemployment, poor physical health, poor mental status, and institutionalization. Yet is is difficult to conceptualize of other populations that cannot be described by these statuses and even more difficult to conceive of other groups susceptible to drug use that cannot be identified by these statuses. Thus, future research should not only attempt to replicate and expand on this model, but should also include populations as subjects of study to ensure the generalizability of the results. Such research should also attempt to demonstrate the direction of causality between status factors and drug use through experimental or longitudinal research designs.

From an applied perspective, the utilization of psychotropic drug use among mentally retarded persons in the present study is quite high for institutionalized persons—9% of adolescents in the community versus 25% of the adolescents in institutions, and 13% of the population in the community versus 35% of the population in institutions. Yet, even within institutions, the observed drug utilization is lower than that cited in the literature. It appears, therefore, that a more conservative approach to their use is currently in practice. Indeed, while the efficacy of psychotropic drugs may be questioned for mentally retarded persons in general (Kirman, 1975; Sprague and Baxley, 1978; JCAH, 1977, Tu, 1979; Murphy, Reagan, and Peterson, 1980), it is particularly questionable for children and youth because their use may further impede learning ability. Thus, many experts (Wolfensberger and Menolascino, 1968; Kirman, 1975; Lipman et al., 1978, Sprague and Baxley, 1978; Silver, 1979; Lipman et al., 1980) caution that a very conservative approach to psychotropic drug use is necessary for mentally retarded children and youth. The results of the present study reflects this admonition in that adolescents in the community and institution are less likely to receive psychotropic drugs than the population. Nonetheless, a further reduction in psychotropic drug use may be appropriate. Other studies have found that psychotropic drugs may be reduced in dosage and often eliminated altogether with no adverse mental or behavior changes by means of behavior therapy programs (Fielding et al., 1980; LaMendola, Zaharia, and Carver, 1980) or by simply using a pharmacist to review medication types and dosages (Inoue, 1982). The status model of drug use would suggest such similar interventions as training in work skills, training in daily living skills, and training in behavior control problems. But much more than that, given these developing skills, the status model emphasizes the need to ensure employment and residential placement in the least restrictive setting. This latter emphasis reflects the fact that while the person may indeed need help, the help should not be limited to psychological or medical props but should include positive changes in the social environment as well.

In sum, from the perspective of the status model, the use of psychotropic drugs is a reactive short-term approach to problems that can be defined as only partially based or blamed on the individual. The use of training for real employment opportunities and for the least restrictive community placement, as well as the simple reduction in use of such drugs, offers a proactive approach that is far more congruent with the long-term goals of individual growth and development in a benign social environment.

## REFERENCE NOTE

1. Janicki, M. P., and Jacobson, J. W. *New York's need assessment and developmental disabilities* (Technical Report, 79 - 10). Albany, N.Y.: New York State Office of Mental Retardation and Developmental Disabilities, 1979.

## REFERENCES

Berg, I., and Hughes, M. Economic circumstances and the entangling web of pathologies: An esquisse. In L. A. Ferman and J. P. Gordus (eds.), *Mental Health and the economy,* Kalamazoo, Mich.: W. E. Upjohn Institute for *Employment Research,* 1979: 15-62.

Berger, P. A. Medical treatment of mental illness. *Science,* 1978, Vol. 200, No. 4344, 974-981.

Brenner, M. H. *Mental Illness and the economy.* Cambridge, Mass: Harvard University Press, 1973.

Dembo, R., Schmeidler, J., and Koval, M. Demographic, Value, and behavior correlates of marijuana use among middle-class youths. *Journal of Health and Social Behavior,* 1976, *17, 2,* 176-186.

DiMascio, A. An examination of actual medication usage in retardation institutions. Portland, Ore: National Meetings of the American Association on Mental Deficiency, 1975.

Fielding, L. T., Murphy, R. T., Reagan, M. W., and Peterson, T. L. An assessment program to reduce drug use with the mentally retarded. *Hospital and Community Psychiatry,* 1980, *31,* 11, 771-773.

Joint Commission on Accreditation of Hospitals. *Standards for services for developmentally disabled individuals.* Chicago: JCAH, 1977.

Inoue, F. A clinical pharmacy service to reduce psychotropic medication use in an institution for mentally handicapped persons. *Mental Retardation,* 1982, *20,* 2, 70-74.

Kirman, B. Drug therapy in mental handicap. *British Journal of Psychiatry,* 1975, 127, 545-549.

LaMendola, W., Zaharia, E. S., and Carver, M. Reducing psychotropic drug use in an institution for the retarded. *Hospital and Community Psychiatry,* 1980, Vol. 31, No. 4, 271-272.

Lipman, R. S. The use of psychopharmacological agents in residential facilities for the retarded. In F. J. Menolascino (ed.), *Psychiatric Approaches to Mental Retardation.* New York: Basic Books, 1970, 387-398.

Lipman, R. S., DiMascio, A., Reatig, N., and Kirson, T. Psychotropic drugs and mentally retarded children. In M. A. Lipton, A. DiMascio, and K. F. Killam (eds.), *Psychopharmacology A Generation of Progress.* New York, Raven Press, 1437-1449, 1978.

Luft, Harold S. Poverty and health: Economic causes and consequences of health problems. Cambridge, Mass: Ballinger Publishing Co., 1978.

Marker, G. Phenothiazines and the mentally retarded: Institutional drug abuse? In Mental Health Law Project, *Mental Health Law Project Summary of Activities,* Washington, D.C., 1975; 1-29.

Sewell, J., and Werry, J. S. Some studies in an institution for the mentally retarded. *New Zealand Medical Journal,* 1976, 84, 317-319.

Silver, L. B. Drug therapy with children and adolescents. In M. J. Cohen (Ed.), *Drugs and the Special Child.* New York: Gardner Press, 1979, 33-62.

Sprague, R. L. and Baxley, G. B. Drugs for behavior management, with comment on some legal aspects. In J. Wortis (ed.), *Mental Retardation: Volume X,* New York: Brunner/Mazel, 1978, 92-129.

Tu, J. B. A survey of psychotropic medication in mental retardation facilities. *Journal of Clinical Psychiatry,* 1979, *40,* 125-128.

Weppner, R. S., Wells, K. S., McBride, D. C., and Ladner, R. A. Effects of criminal justice and mental definitions of a social problem upon the delivery of treatment: The case of drug abuse. *Journal of Health and Social Behavior,* 1976, Vol. 17, No. 2, 170-177.

Wolfensberger, W., and Menolascino, F. J. Methodological considerations in evaluating the intelligence-enhancing properties of drugs. In F. J. Menolascino (ed.), *Psychiatric approaches to mental retardation.* New York: Basic Books, 1979; 399-421.

Zawadski, R. T., Glazer, G. B., and Lurie, E. Psychotropic drug use among institutionalized and noninstitutionalized Medicaid Aged in California. *Journal of Gerontology,* 1978, Vol. 33, No. 6, 825-834.

# Conceptual and Clinical Issues in the Treatment of Adolescent Alcohol and Substance Misusers

## William J. Filstead
## Carl L. Anderson

**ABSTRACT.** This paper describes a system of care and the clinical issues that are central to the delivery of alcoholism and/or substance abuse services to adolescents. Adolescent services can be provided in a variety of settings. Criteria are identified which can distinguish which level of care is most appropriate for the presenting clinical condition of the adolescent.

While the articles in this issue and the references they cite define the extent and scope of adolescent alcohol use and misuse, the relationship of these patterns to adolescent developmental processes, and the clinical thinking that best explains how these problems develop, there are no references to treatment programs and treatment strategies. The treatment of adolescent alcohol and/or substance misusers is an ill-defined topic. In three very significant publications, *Alcohol and Youth: An Analysis of the Literature* (Blane and Hewitt, 1977), *Alcohol and Health, 4th Report to Congress* (1981) and *The Institute of Medicine's Report on Alcohol* (1980), the topic is not even mentioned. The work by Mayer and the senior author (1980) also does not address this topic. Why such a curious

Dr. Filstead is Director of Research and Program Evaluation at the Lutheran Center for Substance Abuse and the Alcoholism Services Division of Parkside Medical Services Corporation. Rev. Anderson is President of Parkside Lodge of Mundelein. Request for copies of this paper should be sent to Dr. Filstead at LCSA, 1700 Luther Lane, Park Ridge, IL 60068.

state of affairs? Given the extensive public pronouncement as to the "epidemic scope" of this problem, the issue of how to treat adolescents with such difficulties is relatively unexplored. Let us provide some suggestive answers:

1. Concern with adolescent alcohol and/or substance misuse developed out of the increasing interest in education, prevention and early intervention programs. It is obvious, so the reasoning goes, that to focus just on treatment issues ignores work that might prevent the development of alcoholism and/or substance misuse in individuals, especially the young.

For a variety of reasons, prevention is thought to be most effective among the youth. While the emphasis has been on prevention, the question of "how to prevent what" is a hotly debated topic (Filstead et al., 1976).

2. When such education and prevention programs began to appear many youth were identified as using alcohol and/or other substances in ways which resulted in a variety of negative social, interpersonal, behavioral, and legal problems. These "problems or troubles" quickly became equated with incipient alcoholism or substance abuse.

While these difficulties and problems were being identified what went unnoticed is that the levels of consumption of alcohol by youth has been essentially stable since World War II (Keller, 1980; Filstead, 1982). The only thing that changed was society's response to this event, not the nature of the event itself. The same behavior a generation apart has been defined differently. However, the use of other substances, especially marijuana is more prevalent among this age group.

3. The topic of adolescence and alcohol/substances contains an array of conceptual and definitional problems. For example, the developmental processes associated with adolescence itself are often ignored, but more likely is not even identified as an issue to consider.

The expectations and perceptions of alcohol and other substances associated with the different age groups that are included in adolescence presents other considerations. In some states 18-year-olds can drink, whereas in others, 21 years of age represents the point where the purchase and consumption of alcohol is legal.

The experimentation with alcohol and/or other substances that is associated with growing up is another consideration. Too frequently data gathered through surveys or structured interviews of nonclinical populations attempts to define a given behavior or a series of experiences as being an indication of abuse. The assumption is that such interpretations are valid. Therefore, the alcoholism and substance abuse field is supposed to develop treatment responses for these identified problems. In effect, nip the bud early before it has a chance to flower into full addiction.

4. What information is known about adolescent use of alcohol and/or other substances comes primarily from surveys of the general population of adolescents. These surveys are often of specific grade levels and/or of community samples. Little data are available on the nature of adolescents who are in treatment. In fact, more is known about the use/misuse and its consequences among non-clinic populations of adolescents than adolescents who are receiving treatment. Curiously, the opposite is true for adults. More is known about treatment populations than the general population of users.

Consequently, what the field believes it understands about adolescent alcohol and/or substance misusers is based on populations who are generally not in treatment. Extrapolations from these survey data are made and then used to indicate the extent and scope of "adolescent alcoholism and/or substance abuse."

In sum, we know very little about the youth who come in contact with alcoholism or substance abuse treatment facilities. Furthermore, the treatment that has been developed for adolescents typically represents a modification of adult treatment programs. It is not surprising that the field starts with what it thinks works, namely how to treat adult alcoholics/substance misusers, and adapts it to fit the adolescents. In many ways this process has prevented the issue of treatment services for the adolescents from being examined in its own right, free from the biases associated with adult programs.

Having tried to provide some tentative answers to why so little literature exists describing adolescents in treatment or the treatment programs for adolescents, the remainder of this paper will concentrate on clinical considerations in the treatment of adolescents. The two general topics that will be explored are: 1) the types of services adolescents need and 2) clinical considerations in delivering such services. The system of care available at the Lutheran Center for Substance Abuse and Parkside Medical Services, Incorporated, members of the Lutheran General Medical Center, forms the basis for the remarks that follow.

## A SYSTEM OF SERVICES

As a starting point, it is useful to consider what types of services adolescent alcohol and/or substance misusers would need. The focus is on what does the patient need rather than what services can a given program offer. Especially with adolescents, a system of care that is available in different settings, which represents varying intensities, that has specific criteria for determining what services in which settings are most appropriate, and is coordinated in order to maximize the "system" nature of care are fundamental principles to the organization and delivery of treatment services for adolescents. What components are the basic elements of such a system?

1. *Evaluation-Assessment Services:* The adolescent and/or family members can present for treatment under varying conditions. The site of initial contact may not be equipped to handle the adolescent. This decision as to the most appropriate treatment setting is made during the initial evaluation-assessment process. The length of time available for evaluation-assessment (E/A) depends upon the presenting clinical condition of the patient. The more acutely distressed the patient (because of either medical and/or psychiatric complications) the shorter the initial E/A time. In any event, should the patient enter treatment the E/A time will occupy the first few days of residential care and/or the first few outpatient visits until a thorough picture of the alcohol/substance abuse along with other concurrent problems are reviewed.

2. *Residential Services:* Many adolescents who reach the point of presenting for help generally have encountered a variety of serious problems in a relatively short span of time. School and/or job performance often is affected. In many cases the adolescent has experienced serious problems in school and may be suspended or expelled. Family relationships are markedly impaired. The legal system often is frequently involved. The presence of other behavior problems and/or psychiatric conditions (e.g., hyperactivity, learning disabilities, mental retardation, violent behavior, suicidal thoughts or gestures, etc.) is not uncommon.

In term of residential services, clinical decisions have to be made as to whether or not residential care is necessary, and if so, what type. Clearly, hospital-based services for acute medical problems are a primary consideration. Such services would be required for patients who present with acute medical problems and/or who develop complications during the detoxification process. While general hospitals can provide such medical technology, the staff often lack an alcoholism/substance abuse perspective. That is why a substance abuse specialty hospital, which can treat the medical and psychiatric problems *concurrent* with alcoholism/substance abuse represents a valuable element in a system of services.

Adolescents who do not manifest the acute medical and/or psychiatric problems can receive treatment in a residential facility. Such a non-hospital program offers a comparable treatment program as the specialty hospital, but lacks the medical staff and intensity of medical services found in the general or substance abuse specialty hospital.

The focus of treatment in a residential setting, be it free standing or specialty hospital based, is to address the misuse of alcohol and/or other substances through educational sessions, group, individual and family sessions, and the reinforcement of positive behavior and the regulations of negative behavior through a peer oriented treatment milieu. It is very important to remember that these patients are *adolescents* as well as substance misusers. Treatment strategies need to address both of these realities.

3. *Outpatient Services:* Outpatient services represent a viable treatment modality. However, it is important to emphasize who is likely to profit from such treatment and something about the approach to take in delivering outpatient services.

The key clinical criteria that would indicate a patient may be a candidate for outpatient services are: 1) absence of acute medical and/or psychiatric problems, 2) ruling out the existence of chronic medical problems that would preclude outpatient treatment, 3) willingness to abstain from all mood altering chemicals, 4) if the person hasn't failed in outpatient treatment in the past, 5) the extent to which the family is interested in becoming involved in the patient's treatment, and 6) the source(s) of motivation. What is behind the person's desire for treatment? If the source of the motivation is strong, regardless of whether or not it is internal, (to stay in school, to make the team, to avoid the jail term, etc.) there is reason to believe outpatient treatment could be considered.

Aside from the evaluation-assessments that are performed on an outpatient basis, for an outpatient program to work there has to be an *intensity of services* which covers a *span of time* during which the concentration and attention is devoted to alcohol/substance misuse and what can be done about it. Once a week sessions do not convey the seriousness of the problem and the treatment commitment that is expected.

Our experience suggests a program of four times per week for four weeks. In addition, the family is expected to participate twice per week, once with the patient as a total family unit and once without the siblings (patient and other children) present. After this primary phase of care the frequency of contact is reduced to twice a week for four weeks. One of these twice a week sessions involves the entire family. The final phase is once a week for twelve weeks.

Throughout the course of this 20 weeks of outpatient treatment there are 36 group sessions, and 12 of the 36 sessions involve the family. Besides the group sessions during the first four weeks, the patient is also seen individually at least once per week. This individual session often precedes a group session. Also, the patient and the parent(s) are expected to actively attend AA and/or NA during the course of treatment.

In operating outpatient services there are a few simple rules that if violated automatically means removal from this level of care with a recommendation for a more restricted treatment setting. In fact, this knowledge that "failing to make it" means a residential treatment referral often acts as a motivating factor for many patients. In order to be involved in outpatient treatment, a few simple rules have to be followed. These rules are: 1) no use of alcohol or other substances for any reason, 2) no violent behavior, 3) regular attendance at therapy sessions, and 4) AA/NA meetings. If the counselor suspects use of substances, a urine screen is requested. Failure to comply results in termination from the program.

4. *Extended Care:* Many adolescents who complete the 4 to 6 weeks of residential care or the 4 to 20 weeks of outpatient treatment still require additional time to continue the rehabilitation process. A return to home or remaining at home may not be the best option for the patient or the family. The change from the structure of residential care to the relative freedom of the home environment is often times too abrupt and dramatic a shift for the adolescent to make. He or she needs to have the time to work at the changes in attitudes and behavior that have been suggested so that they can become more established. Extended care provides a transition period of treatment and re-learning which simulates the responsibilities of daily living but within a structured environment. Obviously, the structure is less than what is experienced during residential treatment, but more than what one would find at home. Residential care focuses intensively

on unlearning old patterns and learning new patterns of behavior in order to accept the need for, and the ability to maintain chemical abstinence. Extended care places an emphasis on putting these skills into practice in everyday living situations. In many outpatient situations, the family environment may not be stable enough to support the patient in his or her home setting and extended care may be the best option to use in responding to this situation.

Extended care can be as short as three months or as long as six months. Patients in this phase of treatment live in a dorm-like setting, each with one other roommate. Patients are expected to be attending school and/or be working. The treatment program is flexible to accommodate the school and/or working schedules of the patients.

In sum, a system of care for adolescents would include: 1) evaluation-assessment capabilities, 2) outpatient services, 3) residential treatment of varying intensity, and 4) extended care services. Not all adolescents need each type of service, but all services are necessary to provide adequate care for adolescents. Furthermore, in each of these settings, there are educational programs of differing format and structure, so that the academic programs of the patients can, as much as possible, be maintained during the course of the treatment.

## CLINICAL CONSIDERATIONS
## IN DELIVERING TREATMENT SERVICES

In developing the system of services described above, a variety of clinical decisions had to be made in shaping both the content of the treatment programs as well as the process of delivering treatment services. These clinical considerations will confront any program that is considering the development of adolescent services. What follows is a discussion of how we responded to them.

1. *Locked Facilities:* The majority of residential treatment occurs at Parkside Lodge, a non-hospital rehabilitation facility. The unit can accommodate up to 40 adolescents in both primary treatment and the evaluation-assessment phase of care. A central concern in opening this program was whether or not a locked unit needed to be part of this facility. Endless discussions occurred for and against the

locked unit. It never was created at the Lodge due primarily to a philosophy of treatment that stressed the individual responsibility of the patient. Having been operational for over 18 months, many professionals have questioned how the facility has been able to operate without a locked unit.

For one, adolescents who could be dangerous to self or others are controlled by the peer pressure/support of the unit. The other adolescents provide the security and support that the physical structure of a locked unit would offer. This is part of the community spirit that the adolescents engender. The fact that human contacts are clearly predominant over external physical controls seems to lessen the desire to act out.

Second, there are occasions (e.g., suicidal ideation, diabetes, medical complications during detoxification, etc.) when adolescents cannot be retained at the Lodge. Most of these patients are referred to the Lutheran Center for Substance Abuse, the specialty hospital. This hospital provides an increased level of medical and psychiatric monitoring and supervision not available at the Lodge. If the patient is in need of a more restrictive environment, the locked psychiatric units of the general hospital are available.

The important point to note is the residential facility functions without a locked unit. Furthermore, there have been no serious incidents that could not be handled by the Lodge. As a result, the extent of acting out behavior, illicit substance use, suicidal gestures, etc., have been controllable. Even though the system of care has the capacity to provide this service, it is not needed at the Lodge. Why?

2. *Clear Expectations:* The principle explanation for this minimal use of locked facilities is the existence of four clearly stated rules, the violation of which results in termination from the program. These four rules are: 1) no alcohol or other drug use, 2) no violence or assaultive behavior, 3) no sexual activity, and 4) no enabling (knowing someone has violated a rule and not informing the community). The adolescents are informed of the importance of these rules. Participation in the program requires compliance with these rules. In order to stay in treatment, adolescents have to comply with these rules. If they break a rule, it is they who have done so and the program simply follows through with the consequences, termination with an appropriate referral.

As the patients perceive these rule violations, the program is not doing something to them; they, the patients, choose to violate the rules. Hence, there is no feeling on their part to act out against the program. Whereas, if the program places the patient in a locked unit, some patients feel something is being done to them and acting out behavior often follows.

These rules are stressed in a variety of ways throughout the detoxification process and the course of treatment. Patients will even comment that no one is really motivated for treatment but that a few are "really not" motivated. These are the individuals who have not accepted the community rules.

3. *Philosophy of Treatment:* A number of points need to be incorporated in an overall philosophy of treatment. The thrust of this philosophy is to convey a clear and consistent message to the patients as to what is expected of them, what treatment consists of and what has to be accomplished if one is to begin a process of recovery.

a. These patients are experiencing the process of adolescence as well as the consequences of alcohol/substance misuse. Staff members need to be aware of this and have an understanding of adolescence per se. Any treatment program which does not address the developmental and identity issues of adolescence will be unsuccessful in engaging the adolescent in treatment.

b. The extent to which misuse of alcohol and/or other substances represents a dependency in this patient population is a much debated topic. So too, is the matter of whether or not these adolescents will be able to drink in their later years. The most appropriate clinical response is to determine the extent to which dependency is present. Dependency is operationally defined to be either increased tolerance and/or physical withdrawal. If such is the case, abstinence is the treatment goal. Even if dependency is not present, but a pattern of repeated difficulties following use exists, abstinence is highly recommended as the treatment goal. Given the extent to which these patients have experienced repeated troubles and difficulties with alcohol and/or other substances, it is unwise to suggest any treatment option other than abstinence.

The adolescents who find their way to treatment are not the kids who get into trouble once or twice when using alcohol or other substances. Adolescents in treatment have a pattern of repeated difficulties, often escalating in seriousness. The treatment premise is simple. If trouble usually occurs with use, it makes no sense to continue using.

c. Often the question is raised about using alcohol in later life.

Again, this is an issue that needs far more investigation. An appropriate response to this concern is to ask the patient to think about why he or she wants to drink? For what purpose? Ultimately only the individual can make this choice. A stress on thinking through the "whys" of the choice to use or not use in later life is far more clinically productive than to say yes or no.

Our advice to patients is to remain chemically free for at least five years and allow themselves the opportunity to develop and grow as individuals. If, after this time, there is still a desire to use alcohol, then the individual needs to weigh this option against his or her past history and the risks that may be associated with a resumption of use.

d. While it is easy to suggest that families need to be a part of the treatment process, this is often a difficult task to accomplish. We choose to address this matter directly. Parents are informed that they are expected to be involved in the treatment of their child. Without their involvement the maximum benefit of treatment may not be achieved and the chances for recovery will be lessened. We express our philosophy of care as one which emphasizes "treatment is not a place." The foundation of a recovery can be laid during treatment, but it has to be built upon in the real world.

In many situations the natural parents are divorced and/or a stepparent may be present. Nevertheless, parental and other family members (siblings) involvement in treatment is vital. One needs to be sensitive to the fact that the climate of the family and the nature of relationships may be less than ideal. Nevertheless, the family needs to be worked with and involved in the patient's treatment.

There are two principle mechanisms for involving the family. The first is through the patient's treatment program. Family members participate in evening lectures and groups, Saturday morning lecture and discussion sessions, and in specified counseling sessions with and without the patient. The second way of involving the family is through a family focused workshop. This three-day workshop attempts to get the family to look at itself apart from the patient. Both of these experiences reinforce each other and the ideas that are being conveyed. Furthermore, both of these experiences stress the value and benefit of Al-Anon, Alateen and Families Anonymous. These self-help groups are an important source of support both during and following the patient's treatment.

4. *Nature of the Treatment Milieu:* Since residential treatment comprises a 4 to 6-week time period, where and how the adolescents live is a very important consideration. There are a few principles which, if followed, can capitalize on this milieu.

a. Physical recreational activities and facilities are essential. These adolescents need an opportunity to run around, work out, "burn off" many sources of frustration and tension. Such activities represent an excellent source of releasing tensions. Furthermore, they provide another arena within which patients and staff can interact.

b. The physical appearance of the unit is important. Paintings, posters, plants, etc., make the unit feel comfortable and inviting. Home-like appearance is the approach that has been used in furnishing the unit. It also provides a feeling of being an enjoyable place to be, but not necessarily a place to stay forever. This sense of comfort also reduces the already existing desire to get out as soon as possible.

If any chair, light fixture, or other object is broken or out of service, it is immediately repaired or replaced. The unit does not have a chance to get run down or appear messy. It is expected that the physical space of the unit will be respected by those who live and work there.

c. Patients are expected to be out of their rooms as much as possible. To promote this goal, no radios or stereos are allowed in the rooms during the first three weeks of treatment. The patient has to earn the privilege of having a radio. A common room contains a TV, stereo, and assorted games. This is the primary gathering place for patients on the unit.

The patients' rooms are to be neat and clean. Beds are to be made and clothes picked up. One visitor made the comment that such standards could not be enforced in a dorm let alone at home. That may very well be, but these standards are enforced in the residential facility. And it is important that they are adhered to since structure and rules are often difficult realities for these adolescents.

d. Similar standards of neatness and cleanliness apply to dress and grooming. The majority of the patients have no difficulty with these standards. Staff initially had more problems than the patients. Staff are expected to dress like professionals, not like adolescents. It needs to be noted that not less, but more structure is helpful with these kids.

## AA Philosophy

The philosophy of AA is very much a part of this treatment system, be it residential or outpatient. The patients have an interesting reaction to the ideas contained within the AA philosophy. Many patients express the point of view that AA provides not only a program that can be followed to achieve recovery, but that AA also provides an explanation for how things got the way they are. In effect, AA provides a framework for helping the patients understand something about themselves as well as put things together vis à vis their alcohol/substance misuse problems.

Many professionals are concerned that by emphasizing the philosophy of AA during this formative period, adolescents will identify with the label of alcoholic as a way of saying who they are. These professionals leave the impression that this identification is at best unwise and at worse unhealthy.

For many of these adolescents, seeing themselves as alcoholic or as a drug abuser would be very healthy whether it be through association with AA or NA or neither. Our experience has been that it is doubtful if any patients should ever try and use again. Of those who will, the prospects for use without problems are very slim. Consequently, seeing oneself as being addicted can be very positive, especially if there are other aspects to their identity aside from the addiction.

The identity of "alcoholic" or "chemically dependent," rather than being a negative stigma is stressed as a positive identity that, once accepted and internalized, brings a sense of freedom to oneself. There are two aspects to this freedom. First, the guilt, anxiety and fear as to what went wrong is reduced by an acceptance of the illness of chemical dependency. Secondly, the person can be free from the predictable impairment in functioning that occurs with the use of mood altering chemicals.

The patients who have participated in AA and/or NA do not see themselves in a unidimensional framework. Perhaps this is the fear professionals have that a strong affiliation with AA or NA would prevent the further growth and development of other aspects of self-identity. Our experience does not support this fear.

## OPERATING AN ADOLESCENT TREATMENT PROGRAM

Having discussed the elements of a system of care and key clinical issues that relate to the delivery of treatment services, it is only appropriate to briefly comment on what one can expect in operating such treatment programs.

First, it is important to select staff who have a capacity to be flexible in their approach to treatment issues. With adolescents it is often important to know when and how far to bend so that the treatment process doesn't break. Many clinical staff do not share the value of "bending." Furthermore, the treatment of adolescents does not take place in a traditional counseling setting, i.e., the hour appointment in the therapist's office. Rather, the therapist has to be out of his or her office spending time with the kids. Spending time often means playing cards, listening to records, talking about "nothing," etc. Such encounters have a significant role to play in generating a sense of trust and in gaining rapport with the adolescents.

Secondly, adolescents present different demands and expectations than adult patients. Staff have to be conscious not to try and fit the adolescents into their way of working with adults. To do so is clinically unproductive and frustrating.

Thirdly, adolescents represent a complex clinical challenge given the developmental processes that are occurring. These issues need to be addressed during the course of treatment. Such matters as sexuality, self-concept, identity crisis, establishing an identity apart from the family, etc., represent issues that alcohol/substance abuse counselors are not generally trained to consider. Furthermore, such concerns are often intertwined with the alcohol and/or substance misuse.

Fourthly, it is important to believe in the value of a thorough evaluation-assessment process through which a determination is made as to the extent of the problem and the appropriate action to take. Far too often adolescents can be misdiagnosed. Rather than prejudging all misuse to be dependency or that no dependency could ever exist among adolescents, it is better to determine exactly what is there. Such a solid foundation is necessary if further treatment is to be successfully employed.

Finally, adolescents may need a variety of services given their clinical condition. One thing is clear about such services. They can be provided in a variety of treatment settings. Therefore, it is imperative to devise criteria and procedures for determining the level of care necessary and the appropriate treatment to provide.

## CONCLUSION

The thrust of this paper has been to emphasize the elements of services that comprise a system of care for adolescent alcohol and/or substance misusers and to identify central clinical considerations that are part of the delivery of treatment services. These areas were addressed in the context of recognizing the importance of adolescence as a developmental process and the implications this poses with respect to the treatment of alcoholism and/or substance misuse.

## REFERENCES

Blane, H., and Hewitt, L. *Alcohol and Youth: An Analysis of the Literature 1960-1975.* Rockville, Maryland: NIAAA, Contract #ADM 281-75-0026. 1977.

*Alcohol and Health: Fourth Special Report to the U.S. Congress.* Rockville, Maryland. NIAAA, 1981.

Mayer, J., and Filstead, W. *Adolescence and Alcohol.* Cambridge: Ballinger Publishing Co., 1980.

Filstead, W., Rossi, J., and Keller, M. (Eds.) *Alcohol and Alcohol Problems: New Thinking and New Directions.* Cambridge: Ballinger Publishing Co., 1976.

*Alcoholism, Alcohol Abuse and Related Problems: Opportunities for Research.* Washington: National Academy Press, 1980.

Filstead, W. "Adolescence and Alcohol." In Pattison, E. M. and Kaufman, E. (Eds.) *Encyclopedic Handbook of Alcoholism.* New York: Gardner Press, 1982, 769-778.

Keller, M. (1980) "Alcohol and Youth" In Mayer, J. and Filstead, W. (Eds.) *Adolescence and Alcohol.* Cambridge: Ballinger Publishing Co., 1980, 245-256.

# Subject Index

Acculturation 77,79,80
Addiction
  intrapsychic 24-26,28-31
  model 32,33
Adolescents
  alcohol intake 1-2
  alcoholic parents of 27-28
  developmental tasks 9-10
  educational needs 12-13
  employment needs 12-13
  parent-oriented 44
  peer-oriented 44
  See also Children
Affection parental 14
Age factors, in drug abuse 77
Age of reason 28
Alcohol abuse
  intake amount 36
  as intrapsychic addiction 24-26
  onset age 36
  parental factors 27-28, 44
  physical factors 27-28
  physiological dependence 24, 25
  prevention 104
  social factors 35
  treatment programs 103-116
    clinical considerations 109-114
  treatment programs
    evaluation-assessment services 106
    extended care 108-109
    family involvement 107,108,112-113
    locked facilities 109-110
    nature of 113-114
    operation of 115
    outpatient services 107-108
    philosophy 111-113
    predominant approach 7
    residential services 106-107, 109-114
    rules 110-111
    shortcomings 24-25

Alcohol use, experimental 36,104-105
Alcoholics Anonymous 25-26,114

Behavioral factors, in substance abuse
  39,53-54
Blacks
  alcohol abuse 61
  divorce rates 60
  drug abuse 57-69
    educational factors 62,64-65
    employment factors 61-62
    family influence 57,59-61,
      62,63,64,65-67
    onset age 58
  drug abuse
    prevention 66-67
    religious factors 64,66
  single parent families 60
  values 64,66
Broken homes 14,59-60

Children
  of alcoholic parents 27-28
  predisposing factors to addiction 23-34
    physical 27-28
    psychological 28-31
    social 31-32
  reasoning processes 28-31
  values 29
Cognitive factors, in substance abuse
  38-39,52-53
Conceptual model, of dependence 2-3
Coping skills deficiency 40-41,59
Correlate research 38-40,51-56,59
Cuban-Americans 73,74,75,77
  See also Hispanics
Cultural factors, in substance abuse 39,
  55-56,79-80

Delinquency 8

   *117*

# Author Index

Abrams, A. 63,64
Aichorn, A. 15
Alibrandi, T. 2
Allen P. 76,77,78
Alpern, S. 16
Amsel, Z. 75,76,77
Assael, M. 16

Ball, J. C. 63,75,76,77
Bannerman, R. 16
Bates, W. M. 60,62,63
Baxley, G. B. 90,91,99
Becker, H. S. 12
Berg, I. 92
Berger, P. A. 90,91
Berkson, R. 16
Blane, H. 103
Bloch, H. W. 13
Bloom, D. 77,82
Bohman, M. 16
Boswell, T. D. 74
Braucht, G. N. 1
Brenner, M. H. 92
Brigance, R. S. 59,64
Brook, J. 60
Brotman, R. 58
Brown, B. S. 60,64,65

Callan, J. P. 58,60
Carolson, J. E. 44
Carver, M. 99
Chambers, C. D. 58,60
Chein, I. 60,61
Clark, R. E. 43
Cloward, R. A. 12
Cohen, A. K. 13
Cooper, D. M. 44
Court-Brown, W. 16
Craig, S. R. 60,64,65
Cressey, D. R. 12
Cullen, R. 74

Crewdson, J. M. 80
Crowther, B. 75,76,77
Culver, C. M. 24
Curtis, B. 75,76
Curtis, R. L. 43

DeFleur, L.B. 72
Delgado, M. 80
Dembo, R. 75,76,77,78,89
DiMascio, A. 90
Dworkin, A. G. 76,79

Edelbrock, C. 44
Edwards, J. 16
Erikson, E. H. 15

Fielding, L. T. 99
Filstead, W. 103,104
Finn, P. 2
Force, E. E. 58
Freedman, A. 58
Friedlander, K. 15

Garcia, J. A. 74
Gert, B. 24
Glaser, D. 58,62,65
Glazer, G. B. 91
Globetti, G. 59,64
Glueck, E. 14
Glueck, S. 14
Glynn, T. J. 59
Goldberg, P. 58
Goldsmith, B. 60
Guinn, R. 75,76,77,78,79

Hagstrom, J. 73,74,75
Halikas, J.A. 58,60,65
Hamburg, B. A. 36
Harford, T. 1
Hays-Bautista, D. E. 81
Hedin, D. 44,59,66